Get-Fit Guy's

Guide to
Achieving
Your Ideal
Body

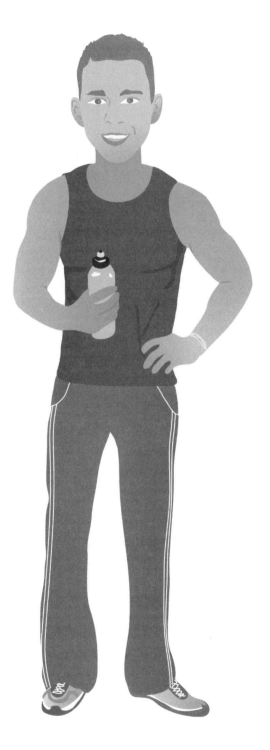

Get-Fit Guy's

Guide to Achieving Your Ideal Body

A Workout Plan
for Your Unique Shape

Ben Greenfield

 St. Martin's Griffin 🐾 New York

IMPORTANT NOTE TO READERS

This book is not intended to replace the advice of your own physician or health-care professional. You should consult a health-care professional before adopting advice concerning diet or exercise or starting a new exercise regimen, especially if you have any existing health problems.

Individual readers are solely responsible for their own health-care decisions. The author and the publisher do not accept responsibility for any adverse effects individuals may claim to experience, whether directly or indirectly, from the information contained in this book.

The fact that an organization or Web site is mentioned in the book as a potential source of information does not mean that the author or the publisher endorse any of the information they may provide or recommendations they may make.

Design by Meryl Sussman Levavi

Library of Congress Cataloging-in-Publication Data

Greenfield, Ben.
  Get-fit guy's guide to achieving your ideal body : a workout plan
for your unique shape / Ben Greenfield. — 1st ed.
      p. cm.
  ISBN 978-1-250-00088-0 (trade paperback)
  ISBN 978-1-250-00912-8 (e-book)
 1. Physical fitness. 2. Exercise. 3. Somatotypes. I. Title.
  RA781.G815
  613.7—dc23
                                                            2012004623

First Edition: May 2012

10 9 8 7 6 5 4 3 2 1

Dedicated to my Mom, who taught me how to write.

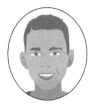

Contents

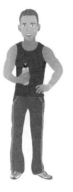

Acknowledgments

The inspiration for this book came from the thousands of readers and listeners of Get-Fit Guy's Quick and Dirty Tips podcast as well as from BenGreenfieldFitness.com. Every day, your honest questions, creative feedback, and committed engagement helped to inspire and motivate me to create this guide to achieving your dream body. Thank you—and if you promise to keep asking questions and sharing your problems, I promise to keep researching answers and finding you solutions!

Thanks to my wife, who is an amazing woman, a superhero mother, a pillar of support, and a warm body for me to hug when I'm stressed out about chapter deadlines or writer's block. I am not sure if I should thank her for cooking, because I probably would have written this book much sooner if I hadn't been pulled away to the dinner table by nightly presentations of aromatic cuisine.

Thanks to my twin boys, River and Terran, who are fully responsible for any typos you may find in this book, as finding the proper letter on a keyboard is more difficult when being attacked by two armed and caped villains who want to engage you in a brutal wrestling match.

Thanks to my parents, who taught me how to read, write, and spell (literally—I was homeschooled), and also served as chaperones and sponsors for tennis, soccer, basketball, running, bicycling, weight lifting, and any other sport I begged to do.

Thanks to Beata Santora, my editor at Quick and Dirty Tips, who kept this ship sailing with countless e-mails and phone calls, and also was patient and gracious enough to put up with my multiple chapter revisions, dumb questions, and strange disappearances for Ironman triathlons. Also thanks to the rest of the team at Quick and Dirty Tips for making possible the weekly Get-Fit Guy audios and articles.

Thanks to all the mentors, coaches, and teachers who have taught me about fitness, nutrition, and healthy living: Dr. Escamilla, Coach Fong, Dr. Dolny, Dr. Browder, Dr. Pearce, Dr. Fitt, Dr. Cohen, Dr. Minkoff, Dr. Dean—this list could go on and on. Please never underestimate the power of sharing your knowledge—it has certainly made a difference in my life.

And thanks to you! You inspire many, many people when you decide to achieve your dream. And I'm one of them.

Get-Fit Guy's

Guide to Achieving Your Ideal Body

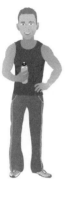

CHAPTER 1

Introduction

Take a look at your ankles. Are they bony? Thick? Muscular? Now move up to your calves. Are they square? Round? Embarrassingly nonexistent?

What about your hips? Are they narrow or curvaceous? As you continue to move up your body, you'll see and feel unique anatomical characteristics that specifically define you, including the shape of your waist and stomach, the breadth of your shoulders, the thickness of your chest, the length of your neck, the size of your wrists, and the roundness of your arms.

Based upon your personal genetics, your fitness, and your health history, your body is unique. Sure, you may have certain characteristics that you've probably noticed on other people too (like broad shoulders or skinny ankles), but life would be pretty boring if we were all identical carbon copies of one another.

And that's not all. Not only is your current body unique, but your *ideal body* is also unique. To understand what I mean, let's try this exercise: Close your eyes and imagine the perfect you. What does that perfect you—your dream body—actually look like? Are your dream body's shoulders broader than your current shoulders? Are your dream body's waist and calves thinner than your current versions? Do your dream body's buttocks fit better into your favorite pair of pants?

Personally, I would prefer less annoyingly bony shoulders, a thicker and more muscular waist, and a more developed backside that might fill out my favorite jeans.

But that's just me.

So whose ideal body is perfect—yours or mine? The answer is neither. Based on the biological individuality of human beings, each of us will have a different shape for our perfect body. Those of us who get fit or lose weight won't finish with identical bodies, and the same is true for those who lose fitness or gain weight.

As a matter of fact, in traditional medical and exercise body typing, also called somatotyping, people are never just skinny or fat. Instead, each of us is placed into one of eight basic body types: female ectomorph, mesomorph, meso-endomorph, and endomorph; and male endomorph, ecto-mesomorph, mesomorph, and endomorph.

Each of these body types has a different basic shape and a different possible ideal body. That's why the perfect shape for one body type simply may not be aesthetically pleasing (or possible) for another body type.

So where did these oddly named categories come from?

We'll have to rewind a few years to go back to the first instance of body typing. Back in the fifth century BC, the philosopher Hippocrates proposed two basic body types, and the Latin phrases he used to describe them can be translated as a long thin body or a short thick body.

More than a thousand years later, in the early 1800s, French physicians began to refer to three different body types: *digestif, musculaire*, and *cerebral*. But body types weren't quantified or described more fully until 1919, when an Italian anthropometrist named Viola took ten measurements of the bodies of a large group of people, compared the individuals to a group average, and came up with three different and difficult-to-pronounce body types, which he quantified and described as:

Microsplanchnic ▷ *small trunk and long limbs, 24 percent of the population*
Macrosplanchnic ▷ *large body and short limbs, 28 percent of the population*
Normosplanchnic ▷ *an intermediate group 48 percent of the population*

A few years later, Ernst Kretschmer, a German psychiatrist, described three body types (and interestingly linked each one to psychiatric problems, which I will conveniently not address in this book). His types were:

Pyknic ▷ *broad, round, and sturdy*
Leptosome ▷ *long and thin, a linear body*
Athletic ▷ *large and muscular thorax and shoulders*

Later, in the 1940s, American psychologist William Sheldon outlined his take on the three basic physiques, using language with which you may be slightly more familiar:

Endomorphic ▷ *spherical body, weak arms, fatty arms and thighs*
Mesomorphic ▷ *broad shoulders and chest, muscled arms and legs*
Ectomorphic ▷ *linear, spindly limbs, narrow chest and abdomen, little muscle and little fat*

Sheldon took his definitions one step further and devised a method of body typing called somatotyping, which was eventually turned into a mathematical model in the late 1960s. In this model, bone length, height-to-weight ratios, fat percentage, photographic analysis, and other measurements were used to develop what is called the Heath-Carter anthropometric somatotype. This model, although very complicated and a real head scratcher if you don't have a math degree, still serves as the basis for scientifically identifying body types.

Of course, most people don't have access to the many tools of measurement and mathematical prowess required for the Heath-Carter anthropometric somatotype method, so you're going to find a far more simple body-typing method within the next few pages of this book.

But first let's delve into a better description of what each body type actually is, since all these "morphisms" can seem confusing. Although I'll give you more detail later on, the lists below briefly illustrate each of the body types for both women and men.

△ *Female Body Types*

Ectomorph   Female ectomorphs are waifish and slim, with thin necks, shoulders, hips, wrists, calves, and ankles—shaped like a ruler. Ectomorphs usually put on weight in their stomach and upper hips, while maintaining slender arms and legs. Taller female ectomorphs tend to be slightly more muscular and are often skilled at endurance sports, but lack the ability to develop curves without the proper exercise program. Gwyneth Paltrow, Thandie Newton, and Kylie Minogue are examples of ectomorphs. Cameron Diaz and Katherine Heigl are taller ectomorphs.

Mesomorph   Female mesomorphs tend to have a classic hourglass shape, with wide shoulders and hips and a distinctively narrow waist. They tend to gain weight and lose weight proportionally in the hips and buttocks, upper back and chest, and have curvy bodies that balance out a bikini top and bottom. A slight weight gain can appear sizable because the mesomorph's body fat easily hides muscle. This type tends to be very athletic and good at a variety of sports and activities. Jessica Simpson, Beyoncé, Scarlett Johansson, Britney Spears, and Jessica Biel are examples of mesomorphs.

Meso-Endomorph   Because of the biological tendency for females to carry more fat than males, female meso-endomorphs are far more common than the male equivalent cross of an ectomorph and mesomorph. They tend to have mid-thickness waists and ankles, small to medium-size shoulders and chests, and wider hips—shaped like a pear. Although out-of-shape meso-endomorphs appear to have a frail upper body with a disproportionately large lower body, they can easily create balance with a proper exercise program. Jennifer Lopez, Elizabeth Hurley, Kim Kardashian, and Minnie Driver are examples of in-shape meso-endomorphs.

Endomorph   Female endomorphs are generally bigger on the top half of their bodies than on the bottom. They commonly have narrow hips and a large chest and stomach, with a curvaceous apple shape. Endomorphs tend to gain weight above the waist or along the buttocks. They are typically good at cardiovascular endurance, but can easily put on weight without a customized exercise and nutrition program. Queen Latifah, Oprah Winfrey, Jennifer Coolidge, and Alex Borstein are examples of endomorphs.

△ *Male Body Types*

Ectomorph   Male ectomorphs have skinny arms and legs; thin waists, wrists, and ankles; and low muscle mass—shaped like a twig. When they do gain weight due to lack of fitness, they put the weight on their stomach and waist. Ectomorphs are often described in the fitness industry as hard-gainers, because they have a tough time building and maintaining muscle mass. However, they usually have a great deal of physical endurance. Clint Eastwood, Ethan Hawke, Billy Bob Thornton, and Chris Rock are examples of ectomorphs.

Ecto-Mesomorphs   Male ecto-mesomorphs can easily fluctuate between being incredibly lean or very muscular. They tend to have broad shoulders; narrow waists, ankles, and wrists; and a V-shaped torso. Like ecto-morphs, when they do gain weight, the fat tends to be on the stomach, but can also be on the buttocks. Ecto-mesomorphs can quickly build muscle and tend to be fairly athletic, but not as power-ful or explosive as mesomorphs (think of a swimmer versus a linebacker). Hugh Jackman, Christian Bale, and Dwayne Wade are examples of ecto-mesomorphs.

Mesomorph   Male mesomorphs are naturally muscular and have a thick, athletic build. They tend to have round, jutting chests, rectangular waists, large arms, thick thighs and calves, and a square shape. Male mesomorphs tend to gain weight easily, especially in the hips, buttocks, upper back, and stomach. Because of their athleticism, mesomorphs respond well to fitness routines and perform well at most physical activities, but must constantly stay active to maintain a fit physique. Russell Crowe, Mark Wahlberg, Dwayne "The Rock" Johnson, Sylvester Stallone, and LL Cool J are examples of mesomorphs.

Endomorph   Male endomorphs are round and typically short (although tall examples, such as Alec Baldwin, do occur). They tend to be curvaceous males with short necks, small shoulders, and thick waists, calves, and ankles—shaped like an apple. Although they tend to have good cardiovascular endurance, endomorphs also have the most difficulty losing weight, and require frequent variations in volume and intensity to maintain fat loss. Seth Rogan, Danny DeVito, Jonah Hill, and Jon Favreau are examples of endomorphs.

You've probably noticed that there are two different combo body types: the female meso-endomorph and male ecto-mesomorph. The reason that the combos for each sex are different is actually quite simple: females are naturally built to carry more fat on their bodies. Don't feel bad, ladies—fat gives you curves, hormones, and perhaps most important, the ability to propagate the human race!

As you can probably imagine, because the body types in the tables above are unique, no single fitness program, workout, exercise machine, number of sets, or cardio class will work ideally for every body type.

For example, a male mesomorph would find himself pretty dissatisfied with his fat-loss progress if he engages in a heavy weight-lifting routine. On the other hand, that very same routine would bestow a toned and curvaceous body upon a female ectomorph. Meanwhile, a female endomorph married to a male endomorph will notice that the long, slow cardio sessions that allow her husband to rapidly shed weight are instead leaving her body frustratingly tired and swollen, and certainly no lighter.

Each body type responds differently to certain workouts and foods and that's where this book comes in.

I'm a personal trainer and a nutritionist. Aside from a brief stint in knee and hip surgical sales, basically all I've done for the past decade is help people get better bodies. I have a folder on my computer of every individual I have personally helped achieve the body of his or her dreams, and that folder contains several thousand individual names. So I've not only seen these eight basic body types over and over again, I've also designed successful individual exercise and meal plans that cater to developing the dream body for each type.

The male endomorph who's been banging his head against the wall trying to shed fat for the past decade? Check.

The female ectomorph who desperately wants some curves so she can fill out her swimsuit? Check.

The former athletes who just can't seem to unlock the secret to getting back the bodies they had in college? Check.

But I didn't simply want to rely on my own experience for writing this book. So for the past two years, I've been running an online survey on my Web site www.bengreenfieldfitness. com. The survey goes into great detail about the characteristics of body shapes, personalities associated with each body shape, meal plans that help each shape achieve the greatest success, and the body parts each shape wants to change the most. The thousands of individual responses and comments on that survey helped tremendously to shape this book—pun intended.

Initially, I didn't set out to write an entire book on this subject. Instead I simply wanted to write an article for my Get-Fit Guy page on the Quick and Dirty Tips network about getting fit for your body type. But having exhaustively studied the types of exercise routines that result in the perfect shape for each type and the specific nutritional regimens that should accompany those routines, I've come to realize that it would take an entire book to contain the knowledge necessary to figure out your body type and achieve your ideal body using a customized workout.

So the bottom line is that this book that you're holding in your hands or looking at on your e-book reader or perhaps even scrolling through on your smartphone comes from over a decade of experience in body identification and transformation and from the responses of thousands of people just like you. The underlying principle of this book is that by identifying your unique body type and performing a fitness routine specifically designed for that shape, you can achieve your ideal physical appearance—*your ideal body.*

That's right, this book is going to find your ideal body and give it to you!

Here's how it works:

First, you'll easily identify your body type using a step-by-step self-typing system, which is what you'll find in the first part of this book. If you'd prefer a digital version, you can access these same questionnaires at GetFitGuy.com where I've also included a host of convenient resources to accompany this book. And that's great news—because it means that identifying your body type will not require expensive laboratory visits, needles, muscle biopsies, bloodletting, or complicated math (although you will need to measure a few body parts, sorry!).

Next, once you have identified your body type, you'll learn the specific anatomical changes in your ankles, calves, hips, thighs, butt, waist, chest, shoulders, arms, wrists, and neck that will allow you to achieve your dream body. You'll also be given a fitness system and workout routine to make those changes. And even though this isn't a diet book per se, you'll also receive body shape–specific nutrition advice to help you with meal planning and dietary changes to transform your current shape into your ideal body.

After that, you just sit back and wait.

Just kidding!

Then you'll head to the gym armed with your easy-to-understand workout plan, to the grocery store to fill your kitchen with the foods you'll need to change your diet, and to the Get-Fit Guy Facebook page* to ask me any questions you have along the road toward your dream body.

Sounds like a plan? Fantastic.

Let's get started with your body-type questionnaire.

* Facebook.com/getfitguy

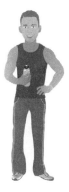

CHAPTER 2

Female Body-Typing Questionnaire

Are you ready to find out which of the four body types you are? This questionnaire will ask you about your physical attributes, diet tendencies, and lifestyle, and will allow you to quickly and accurately pinpoint your body type!

As you read through each item, simply choose the answer that best describes you. Usually that's the answer that comes to mind first.

There are some questions that ask you about what happens when you exercise, when you lose or gain weight, when you're healthy or when you don't eat healthfully. *If you're unsure about an item or it doesn't apply to your unique situation, simply leave the question unanswered and move on.*

For items 10 and 16, you'll want a flexible measuring tape that you can wrap around a body part.

You can also take this questionnaire online at GetFitGuy .com/questionnaires.

1. Physical Attributes

1. For my body size, my feet are:
   a. Large.
   b. Medium.
   c. Small.

2. When I stand in place or walk, my feet tend to:
   a. Point in (pigeon-toed).
   b. Point forward.
   c. Point out (duck walk).

3. My lower calves and upper ankles are:
   a. Skinny, with visible bones and veins.
   b. Shapely, somewhat muscular.
   c. Thick, without a significant decrease in size from calf to ankle.

4. My upper calves are:
   a. Thin, without much muscle. I have a hard time putting muscle on them.
   b. Defined and can bulk up when I exercise.
   c. Bulky or curvaceous. They may cramp when I'm exercising.

5. My thighs:
   a. Are narrow, without a significant taper from hip to knees.
   b. Are muscular and/or gain muscle quickly, but also tend to be fat magnets.
   c. Are cylindrical and round, with some cellulite.

6. My hips are:
   a. Not very different in width than my torso and waist.
   b. Curvy, markedly wider than my waist.
   c. Narrower than my upper body.

7. If I measure the narrowest part of my waist and the widest part of my hips, then divide the waist number by the hip number, my waist:hip ratio is:
   a. Less than 0.7.
   b. 0.7 to 0.8.
   c. Greater than 0.8.

8. My stomach is:
   a. Flat, but it's the place where excess weight gain occurs.
   b. Strong and firm. If I gain weight, it concentrates on my hips rather than my stomach.
   c. Curvy, even if I'm in good shape.

9. My breasts are:
   a. A–B cup.
   b. C–D cup.
   c. D+ cup.

10. My back is:
    a. Narrow and straight, without much of a width change from behind the armpits down the waist.
    b. V-shaped, tapering from the upper back down to the waist.
    c. Wider on the bottom (near the hips) than on top (at the shoulders).

11. My shoulders are:
    a. Thin and narrow, with a tendency toward injury or rotator cuff problems.
    b. Broad and square, where I tend to easily build muscle.
    c. Smaller than the rest of my upper body.

12. If I compare my shoulders to my hips:
    a. They are the same width.
    b. My shoulders are wider than my hips.
    c. My hips are wider than my shoulders.

13. My arms are:
    a. Skinny, with visible veins.
    b. Muscular, but tend to gain weight in the upper arms.
    c. Thick, without much muscle definition.

14. If I measure around the smallest part of my wrist, it is:
    a. 5.5 to 5.99 inches.
    b. 6 to 6.25 inches.
    c. Greater than 6.25 inches.

15. When I wrap my thumb and middle finger around my wrist:
    a. My fingers overlap.
    b. My fingers touch.
    c. My fingers do not touch.

16. My hands are:
    a. Long, with skinny fingers.
    b. Long, but fingers are shorter with square ends.
    c. Short and small.

17. My face is:
    a. Oval-shaped.
    b. Square or heart-shaped.
    c. Round or rectangle-shaped.

18. My height is:
    a. Less than 5 feet 3 inches (157 cm).
    b. More than 5 feet 8 inches (174+ cm).
    c. 5 feet 3 inches to 5 feet 8 inches (160–173 cm)

19. I have:
    a. No cellulite.
    b. Some cellulite on my upper legs and butt.
    c. Significant cellulite on my lower body.

20. If I gain weight, the first place on my body it goes to is:
    a. My middle.
    b. My butt and upper legs.
    c. All over evenly, even to my hands and feet.

21. If I start eating poorly and not exercising:
    a. I don't gain a significant amount of weight.
    b. I gain weight quickly but can lose it rapidly.
    c. I gain weight quickly and have a hard time losing it.

22. My figure is best described by these proportions (bust-waist-hips):
    a. 34-30-35, 36-33-37, or 40-36-42.
    b. 32-26-33, 33-27-35, or 36-30-38.
    c. 40-36-33, 36-32-30, or 34-30-29.

2. Lifestyle

23. If I weight train:
    a. I have a hard time putting on muscle or getting stronger.
    b. I bulk up and add strength quickly.
    c. I get stronger, but have a hard time seeing muscle definition.

24. When it comes to diet and nutrition:
    a. I am hungry all the time and feel like constantly snacking.
    b. I feel fine on three square meals a day.
    c. It seems like I can go all day without eating.

25. When I go to the doctor for a physical with blood work, I tend to have:
    a. Low fasting blood sugar.
    b. Normal to midrange fasting blood sugar.
    c. High fasting blood sugar.

26. My family history of diabetes is:
    a. No one in my family has it.
    b. Some distant family members have it.
    c. My parents, siblings, or other close relatives have it.

27. When it comes to food, I crave:
    a. Sweet and starchy carbohydrates (like cookies or candy).
    b. Rich and spicy foods (like tacos or Indian food).
    c. Dairy products, or greasy, salty foods (like chips or hamburgers).

28. For coffee or caffeinated drinks, each day I have:
    a. 0–1 cups.
    b. 2–3 cups.
    c. More than 3 cups.

Add up your a responses and write the total here: _____
Add up your b responses and write the total here: _____
Add up your c responses and write the total here: _____

If you have 20 or more *a* responses, you are an ectomorph.
If you have 20 or more *b* responses, you are a mesomorph.
If you have 20 or more *c* responses, you are an endomorph.

If you do not have 20 responses in any category, but your *b* and *c* responses combined total 20 or more, then you are a meso-endomorph.

Once you've completed the questionnaire, these body-type illustrations and underlying descriptions will help you visualize the four different female body types.

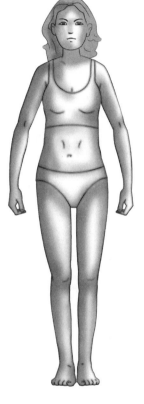

Female ectomorphs are waif-like and slim, with thin necks, shoulders, hips, ankles, wrists, and calves—shaped like a ruler. When out of shape, ectomorphs tend to put on weight in their stomach and upper hips, while maintaining slender arms and legs. Taller female ectomorphs tend to be slightly more muscular and are often skilled at endurance sports, but lack the ability to develop curves without the proper exercise program. A perfect example of a distinction between an ectomorph and the next body type (meso-morph) is Venus and Serena Williams. Venus is an ecto-morph, while her sister Serena is a mesomorph.

Celebrity Ectomorphs
Gwyneth Paltrow
Thandie Newton
Kylie Minogue
Cameron Diaz
Kristen Stewart

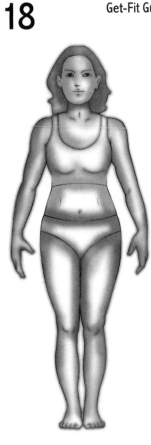

Female mesomorphs tend to have a classic hourglass shape, with wide shoulders and hips and a distinctively narrow waist. They tend to both gain weight and lose weight proportionally in the hips and buttocks, upper back, and chest, and have curvy body types that tend to balance out a bikini top and bottom. When a mesomorph puts on just a little weight, it appears like a large gain because their body fat easily hides muscles. Because of their naturally high amount of lean muscle and V-shaped body, mesomorphs tend to be very athletic and good at a variety of sports and activities.

Celebrity Mesomorphs

Jessica Simpson

Beyoncé Knowles

Scarlett Johansson

Serena Williams

Jennifer Garner

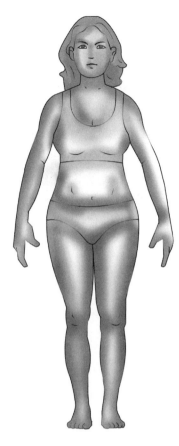

Female meso-endomorphs are far more common than the male equivalent cross of an ectomorph and mesomorph. They tend to have mid-thickness waists and ankles, small to medium-size shoulders, smaller chests, somewhat narrow waists, with fairly wide hips, buttocks, and thighs—a pear shape. Although out-of-shape meso-endomorphs appear to have a frail upper body with a disproportionately larger lower body, they can balance this tendency with a proper exercise regimen—and even become *People* magazine's most beautiful woman.*

Celebrity Meso-Endomorphs

*Jennifer Lopez**
Minnie Driver
Kim Kardashian
Anna Kournikova
Halle Berry

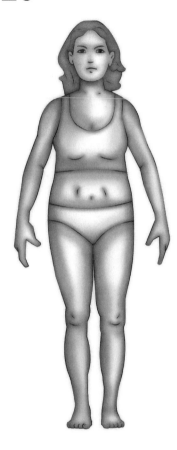

Female endomorphs are generally bigger on the top half of their bodies than on the bottom half. They commonly have slim hips and a large chest and torso, with a curvaceous apple shape. Although they can sometimes have thick calves and ankles, endomorphs tend to gain weight above the waist or along the buttocks. They are typically good at cardiovascular endurance, but can easily gain weight without a customized exercise and nutrition program.

Celebrity Endomorphs
Queen Latifah
Oprah Winfrey
Jennifer Coolidge
Kate Winslet

In addition to the body typing questionnaire, if you visit GetFitGuy.com, you can have free access to a body-fat calculator, a body-frame calculator, and an ideal-weight calculator—all of which will help you track your progress and measure your body even more efficiently.

Now that you know your body type, it's time for the fun to begin. Simply turn to the chapter for your body type and begin learning the specific exercises, workouts, and dietary approach that is going to get you your dream body!

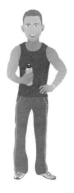

CHAPTER 3

Male Body-Typing Questionnaire

Are you ready to find out which of the four body types you are? This questionnaire will ask you about your physical attributes, diet tendencies, and lifestyle, and will allow you to quickly and accurately pinpoint your body type!

As you read through each item, simply choose the answer that best describes you. Usually that's the answer that comes to mind first.

There are some questions that ask you about what happens when you exercise, when you lose or gain weight, when you're healthy or when you don't eat healthfully. *If you're unsure about an item or it doesn't apply to your unique situation, simply leave the question unanswered and move on.*

For items 7 and 14, you'll want a flexible measuring tape that you can wrap around a body part.

You can also take this questionnaire online at GetFitGuy .com/questionnaires.

1. Physical Attributes

1. For my body size, my feet are:
   a. Large.
   b. Medium.
   c. Small.

2. When I stand in place or walk, my feet tend to:
   a. Point in (pigeon-toed).
   b. Point forward.
   c. Point out (duck walk).

3. My lower calves and upper ankles are:
   a. Thin, with visible bones and veins.
   b. Shapely, somewhat muscular.
   c. Thick, without a significant decrease in width from calf to ankle.

4. My upper calves are:
   a. Thin, without much muscle. I have a hard time putting muscle on them.
   b. Are medium sized and bulkier toward the top. If I exercise regularly, they can get very defined.
   c. Round or curvaceous. They may cramp when I'm exercising.

5. My thighs:
   a. Are narrow, without a significant taper from hip to knees.
   b. Are muscular toward the top, but get thinner toward the knees.
   c. Are thick and round from thigh to knee.

6. My hips are:
   a. Narrower than my waist.

    b. About the same width as my waist.

    c. Wider than my waist.

7. If I measure the narrowest part of my waist and the widest part of my hips, then divide the waist number by the hip number, my waist-to-hip ratio is:

    a. Less than 0.9.

    b. 0.9 to 1.0.

    c. Greater than 1.0.

8. My stomach is:

    a. Flat, but it's the place where I notice excess weight gain.

    b. Strong and firm. If I gain weight, it concentrates on the sides of my waist or on my lower body rather than on the front of my stomach.

    c. Round.

9. My chest is:

    a. Narrow or flat.

    b. Square or muscular.

    c. Barrel-shaped or round.

10. My back is:

    a. Narrow and straight, without much of a width change from behind the armpits down the waist.

    b. V-shaped, tapering from the upper back down to the waist.

    c. Wider on the bottom (near the hips) than on top (at the shoulders).

11. My shoulders are:

    a. Thin and narrow, with a tendency toward injury or rotator cuff problems.

    b. Broad and square, where I tend to easily build muscle.

    c. The same width or smaller than the rest of my upper body.

12. If I compare my shoulders to my hips:
    a. My shoulders are slightly wider than or the same size as my hips.
    b. My shoulders are significantly wider than my hips.
    c. My hips are wider than my shoulders.

13. My arms are:
    a. Skinny, with visible veins.
    b. Muscular, and tend to easily gain mass.
    c. Thick, without much muscle definition.

14. If I measure around the smallest part of my wrist, it is:
    a. 5.5 to 6.5 inches.
    b. 6.6 to 7.5 inches.
    c. Greater than 7.5 inches.

15. When I wrap my thumb and middle finger around my wrist:
    a. My fingers overlap.
    b. My fingers touch.
    c. My fingers do not touch.

16. My hands are:
    a. Long, with skinny fingers.
    b. Long, but fingers are shorter with square ends.
    c. Short and thick.

17. My jaw is:
    a. Thin and pointy, like Johnny Depp.
    b. Square with a well-defined chin, like Sylvester Stallone.
    c. Round but relatively narrow, like Jack Black.

18. My height is:
    a. Less than 5 feet 7 inches (170 cm).
    b. More than 5 feet 10 inches (178+ cm).
    c. 5 feet 7 inches to 5 feet 9 inches (170–182 cm).

19. If I gain weight, the first place on my body it goes to is:
    a. My stomach.
    b. My butt, upper legs, or love handles.
    c. All over evenly, even to my hands and feet.

20. If I start eating poorly and not exercising:
    a. I don't gain a significant amount of weight.
    b. I gain weight quickly but can lose it rapidly.
    c. I gain weight quickly and have a hard time losing it.

2. Lifestyle

21. If I weight train:
    a. I have a hard time putting on muscle or getting stronger.
    b. I bulk up and add strength quickly.
    c. I get stronger, but have a hard time seeing muscle definition.

22. If I run, I am:
    a. Good at jogging quickly for long periods of time.
    b. Good at fast running efforts of less than 2 minutes.
    c. Good at powerful, explosive sprints and at jogging slowly.

23. When it comes to diet and nutrition:
    a. I am hungry all the time and feel like constantly snacking.
    b. I feel fine on three square meals a day.
    c. It seems like I can go much of the day without eating.

24. When I go to the doctor for a physical with blood work, I tend to have:
    a. Low fasting blood sugar.
    b. Normal to midrange fasting blood sugar.
    c. High fasting blood sugar.

25. My family history of diabetes is:
    a. No one in my family has it.
    b. Some distant family members have it.
    c. My parents, siblings, or other close relatives have it.

26. When it comes to food, I crave:
    a. Sweet and starchy carbohydrates (like cookies or candy).
    b. Rich and spicy foods (like tacos or Indian food).
    c. Dairy products, or greasy, salty foods (like chips or hamburgers).

27. For coffee or caffeinated drinks, each day I have:
    a. 0–1 cups.
    b. 2–3 cups.
    c. More than 3 cups.

Add up your a responses and write the total here: _____
Add up your b responses and write the total here: _____
Add up your c responses and write the total here: _____

If you have 19 or more *a* responses, you are an ectomorph.
If you have 19 or more *b* responses, you are a mesomorph.
If you have 19 or more *c* responses, you are an endomorph.

If you do not have 19 responses in any category, but your *a* and *b* responses combined total 19 or more, then you are an ecto-mesomorph.

Once you've completed the questionnaire, these body-type illustrations and underlying descriptions will help you visualize the four different male body types.

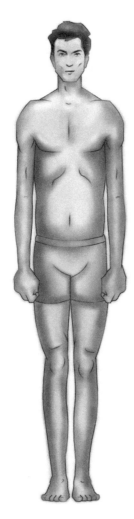

Male ectomorphs have skinny arms and legs; thin waists, wrists, and ankles; low muscle mass; and twig or stick shapes. When an ectomorph gains weight due to lack of fitness, he puts the weight on his stomach and waist. Ectomorphs are often described in the fitness industry as hard-gainers because they have a hard time building and maintaining muscle mass, although they usually have a great deal of physical endurance.

Celebrity Male Ectomorphs
Clint Eastwood
Ethan Hawke
Billy Bob Thornton
Chris Rock

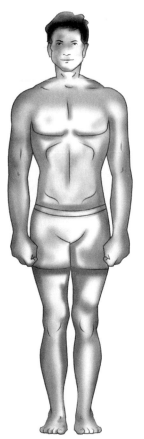

Male ecto-mesomorphs can easily fluctuate between being incredibly lean and being very muscular. They tend to have broad shoulders; narrow waists, ankles, and wrists; and a V shape. Like ectomorphs, when they do gain weight, the fat tends to be on the stomach, but can also be on the buttocks. Like mesomorphs, the next body type, they can quickly build muscle and tend to be fairly athletic, but not as powerful or explosive (think of a swimmer versus a linebacker).

Celebrity Male Ecto-Mesomorphs

Hugh Jackman
Christian Bale
Dwayne Wade
Ben Greenfield

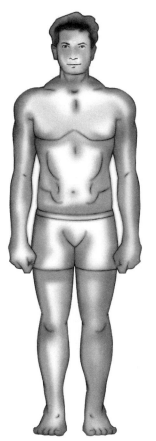

Male mesomorphs are naturally muscular and have a thick, athletic build. They tend to have round, jutting chests, rectangular waists, large arms, thick thighs and calves, and a square shape. However, male mesomorphs tend to gain weight easily, especially in the hips, buttocks, upper back, and stomach. Because of their athleticism, mesomorphs respond well to fitness routines and perform well at most physical activities, but must constantly stay active to maintain a nice body.

Celebrity Male Mesomorphs

Mark Wahlberg

Dwayne "The Rock" Johnson

Sylvester Stallone

Bruce Willis

LL Cool J

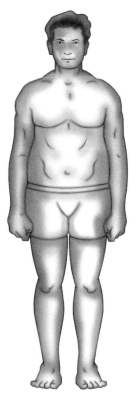

Male endomorphs are round and typically short (although there are tall examples, such as Alec Baldwin). They tend to be curvaceous males with short necks; narrow shoulders; thick waists, calves, and ankles; and a round apple shape. Although they tend to have good cardiovascular endurance, endomorphs also have the most difficulty losing weight, and require frequent variations in volume and intensity to maintain fat loss.

Celebrity Male Endomorphs

Seth Rogan
Jonah Hill
Danny DeVito
Jon Favreau
Russell Crowe

In addition to the body typing questionnaire, if you visit GetFitGuy.com, you can have free access to a body-fat calculator, a body-frame calculator, and an ideal-weight calculator—all of which will help you track your progress and measure your body even more efficiently.

Now that you know your body type, it's time for the fun to begin. Simply turn to the chapter for your body type and begin learning the specific exercises, workouts, and dietary approach that is going to get you your dream body!

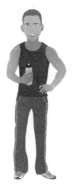

CHAPTER 4

Body Type: Female Ectomorph

This may make you sound like some kind of delicate dinner cracker, but the female ectomorph body is often described as "waiflike." And although you're not necessarily as fragile as this description makes you seem, you are definitely the thinnest of the female body types. You have low amounts of both fat and muscle, and are slim with small and narrow shoulders, chest, hips, and buttocks. You also tend to have skinny ankles, wrists, and calves, and a thin neck. This combination of characteristics tends to give you a linear, "ruler" shape. Of course, it is possible for that ruler to slightly change, and when out of shape, you mostly put weight on your stomach and upper hips, while maintaining those slender arms and legs. Although this may make you grimace, this is often referred to as the "skinny-fat" look. Sorry—not my invention!

Gwyneth Paltrow, Paula Radcliffe, Thandie Newton, and

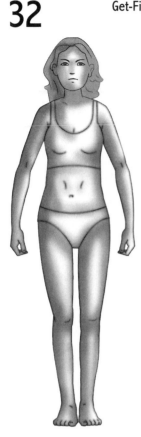

Kylie Minogue are examples of typical ectomorph bodies. Taller female ectomorphs, like Cameron Diaz and Katherine Heigl, tend to be slightly more muscular, but even they lack the ability to develop significant curves without the proper exercise program. Interestingly, just because you have an ectomorph body does not mean you come from a family of ectomorphs. A perfect example of this type of familial distinction between an ectomorph and the next body type are tennis players Venus and Serena Williams. Venus is closest to an ectomorph body type, while her sister is a definite mesomorph.

Your Strengths

Because you are naturally thin, with low body fat and an efficient metabolism, you can eat more without gaining significant amounts of weight, and this may sometimes make your non-ectomorph friends jealous—especially when the bread, chips, and cookies that cause them to balloon are relatively risk-free for you from the standpoint of weight gain.

Your body type tends to be superior at endurance sports, because you can burn fat efficiently, stay cool due to your low body mass, and move for long periods of time without getting tired. Your light weight and graceful appearance also means you are likely to excel at (or be drawn to) sports such as dance or ice-skating.

Although you may fear that your shape can appear boyish, this is not really the case, as many beautiful female supermodels (think Kate Moss) actually have your same classic long, slender ectomorph shape. However, if your natural skinniness bothers you, not only can the right exercise program help, but you will also get more curvaceous (or gain weight) with age as your naturally high metabolism begins to slow. While you may enjoy having a curvier shape at first, this natural weight gain can also cause significant fat formation on your stomach and buttocks—especially if you don't exercise or if you continue to eat whatever you want—so be careful!

However, regardless of age, you probably don't have to worry about fat arms and legs, and it can be very easy for you to tone these areas with a proper workout program. In addition, as you lift weights to get the lean muscle that will allow you to achieve your dream body, you don't need to worry about your body type bulking up or getting too muscular. Looking like an estrogen-enhanced version of Incredible Hulk just isn't a possibility for a female ectomorph.

Your Limitations

As you know, it can be a struggle to attain a more curvaceous appearance or fill out your clothes. You tend to lack these curves due to your low muscle mass, low body fat, and small frame. In addition, low muscle mass and a small frame means that certain joints and muscle groups can be weak—and the last nickname you want is "skinny slouch"!

You will find that compared with other body types, you produce less force, especially when it comes to weight training or playing sports that require strength or power. At the same time, these are the precise activities that will help you build bone mass and avoid osteoporosis as you age. For this reason, it is extremely important for you to engage in weight-bearing activities like weight lifting or explosive activities like fast running, even if they're more difficult for your body type.

Because you have a high metabolism that uses lots of calories, exercise such as the workout plan in this book may result in muscle breakdown and loss unless you rest and recover between workouts. You also need to focus on post-workout nutrition by replenishing carbohydrates and proteins. But don't get too carried away with your daily food intake! Since your metabolism is so high, you may find it difficult to control cravings for junk food, and even though excess carbohydrates won't cause excessive weight gain if you are exercising, too many starches and sugars can increase your risk of cardiovascular disease and diabetes.

Your Ideal Body

Remember that the female ectomorph body is often seen in supermodels and dancers, and your long arms and legs and linear physique can actually work to your advantage if you use the appropriate workout program to add lean, defined muscle. Weight training is absolutely crucial to this goal, but compared to the other body types, your natural leanness allows you to easily develop a firm, toned physique. Your low body fat means that each fiber of muscle that you add to your body will result in tight definition in your arms and legs, a flat stomach with visible muscle lines, and firm upper body curves.

Even though your thighs, hips, and rear are relatively small compared to other body types, they will also respond well to weight training, and can easily develop curves that accentuate your toned arms and legs. With the exercises in this chapter for your upper hips, stomach, butt, and lower back, you can develop a functional and firm core that makes the connection between your upper and lower body look very defined and athletic. If you open the pages of any running magazine, you can see that many female runners have such a flat stomach.

To see examples of well-formed female ectomorph body shapes, do an internet search or look in magazines for images of Kate Moss, Audrey Hepburn, Cameron Diaz, Thandie Newton, Lisa Kudrow, Nicole Kidman, Goldie Hawn, and Gisele Bundchen.

Your Workout Plan

As a female ectomorph, you should restrict your amount of cardiovascular exercise. Even though it can be difficult to avoid this type of exercise, especially since you're naturally gifted at long, slow efforts, the problem is that such exercise burns calories without adding lean muscle fiber—and thus will contribute to a frail, nonmuscular appearance. Those female ectomorph runners I mentioned earlier aren't just pounding countless miles on the pavement; they're doing lots of weight training and core exercise to ensure they stay injury-free and don't become frail or gaunt.

The other issue with long bouts of cardio is that you'll have to figure out a way to eat significant amounts of extra food to replace all those calories you're burning, which can be stressful for you and your body's hormones and metabolism. This is one reason that women who only do big bouts of cardiovascular exercise can have hormonal imbalances and immune-system deficiencies.

So unless you are training very seriously for a marathon or triathlon, you should spend the majority of your exercise time performing resistance-training workouts with weights, which will allow you to increase lean muscle and add curves. Unlike the curves you'll develop from simply eating more food and increasing your fat stores, the curves from weight training will be firm and defined (not to mention healthier!). You're not completely banned from doing cardiovascular exercise, but these workouts should be limited to just two to three short, high intensity cardio intervals each week, and there is no need for these sessions to last any longer than 30 minutes (unless you're bumping up to half-marathons and beyond).

When you perform your weight training workouts, you need to choose heavy weights and perform a low number of repetitions. To maximize the rate at which you add lean muscle and the beneficial, muscle-defining hormonal response to your weight training sessions, most of the exercises should be multi-joint compound exercises that involve more than one muscle group. A squat is one such exercise, while a machine leg extension is not.

Below, I've designed a female ectomorph workout that should ideally be performed three to four days per week, with at least 24 hours of recovery between each workout. This plan is designed to increase lean, toned muscle and curves—and incorporates back-to-back supersets for opposing muscle groups, with no rest between sets so that you can maximize your time at the gym. Yes, this means you won't be spending much time sitting and reading magazines during your weight training! Save the socializing for your cool-down.

If this workout seems like an impossible chunk of time or effort for you and you want to lift weights for a shorter period of time, you can easily adapt the workout to do shorter, more frequent sessions. You can do this by performing supersets 1 and 2 on the first day, supersets 3 and 4 on the next day, inserting one day of rest, and then repeating for three additional days of the week. Don't worry—if any of that seems confusing, you can just head over to Facebook.com/GetFitGuy and ask your questions! Just remember that any time you're overwhelmed with exercise, doing a little bit is better than doing nothing at all.

Even though heavier lifting is required to add curves to your ectomorph body, one likely consequence of choosing heavier weights is the likelihood that your muscles will fatigue before you achieve the recommended number of repetitions. So if you cannot complete a set using the weight you've chosen for an exercise, stop, rest a few seconds, and then keep going, rather than just decreasing to an easier weight. As a personal trainer, I've found that female ectomorphs are notorious for choosing light weights and simply lifting that weight for very long periods of time. That's not how to get your dream body!

Finally, you'll notice that there are alternative movements to each of the exercises. Since you should ideally be switching up your workouts every four to six weeks, these will come in handy. To see examples of alternative pushing, pulling, rowing, twisting, extending, and other exercises, simply visit GetFitGuy.com/exercises.

For a detailed explanation of sets, reps, tempo, load, and other weight training tips, go to "Definitions" in the Appendix (p. 135). You can print workouts to take to the gym with you at GetFitGuy.com.

△ *Female Ectomorph Full Body Workout*

Exercise	Sets	Reps	Tempo	Load
Warm-up: Complete 3–5 minutes of aerobic exercise such as jogging, cycling, or using an elliptical trainer. Or complete the warm-up program in the Appendix of this book (p. 141).				
Superset 1: Complete the following exercises back to back with minimum rest. Rest 60–90 seconds, then repeat, for 2–5 sets. Beginners should choose a lower range of sets, while more advanced exercisers can do the higher range.				
Alternating overhead presses, **p. 205**	2–5	8–10	fluent	80–85%
Seated rows, **p. 234**	2–5	8–10	fluent	80–85%
Superset 2: Complete the following exercises back to back with minimum rest. Rest 60–90 seconds, then repeat, for 2–5 sets.				
Stability ball chest presses, **p. 228**	2–5	8–10	fluent	80–85%
Pull-ups or pull-downs, **p. 242**	2–5	8–10	fluent	80–85%
Superset 3: Complete the following exercises back to back with minimum rest. Rest 60–90 seconds, then repeat, for 2–5 sets.				
Dumbbell or barbell squats, **p. 211**	2–5	8–10	fluent	80–85%
Romanian dead lifts, **p. 217**	2–5	8–10	fluent	80–85%

EXERCISE	SETS	REPS	TEMPO	LOAD
Superset 4: Complete the following exercises back to back with minimum rest. Rest 60–90 seconds, then repeat, for 2–5 sets. You can choose any flexing/extending exercises for the lower body.				
Cable torso twist, **p. 230**	2–5	8–10	fluent	80–85%
Water-ski row, **p. 231**	2–5	8–10	fluent	80–85%
Cool-down: Finish with 3–5 minutes of light aerobic activity such as cycling or brisk walking, followed by a full body stretch. Visit Tinyurl.com/benstretch for a full body-stretching protocol.				

On the days that you are not weight training, you can perform the following optional cardio interval workouts on a bicycle, treadmill, elliptical trainer, rowing machine, or walking or running outdoors. These are entirely optional, and if your time is limited, you should prioritize the weight training, since your body is already naturally good at cardiovascular exercise, and you may have a hard time adding curves, muscles, or weight if you overdo the cardio.

The only reason you would need to include the cardio intervals is if you are training for a 5K, half-marathon, or other endurance event, or if you huff and puff every time you climb a flight of stairs and want to include a bit of extra cardio. Although I hesitate to say this, because I've seen many female ectomorphs do well in events such as Ironman triathlons and marathons with primarily weight training and intense cardio intervals, you need to add in at least one day of long, slow cardio if you plan on doing very long endurance events.

If you are weight training every day, then you can either use these cardio workouts as a warm-up for your weight training or do them at a separate time of day—but unless you fit the criteria above, do not include cardio interval training more than three days per week.

High Intensity Cardio Interval Workout 1

5-minute warm-up (jumping jacks, running in place, cycling, elliptical, rowing)

4 minutes at the highest effort you can sustain

4 minutes at a moderate pace

3 minutes at the highest effort you can sustain

3 minutes at a moderate pace

2 minutes at the highest effort you can sustain

2 minutes at a moderate pace

3-minute cool-down

High Intensity Cardio Interval Workout 2

5 minutes at a moderate pace

1 minute as hard as possible, followed by 1 minute at a moderate pace

2 minutes as hard as possible, followed by 1 minute at a moderate pace

3 minutes as hard as possible, followed by 1 minute at a moderate pace

Repeat steps 2–4

2-minute cool-down

High Intensity Cardio Interval Workout 3

5 minutes at a moderate pace

3×30 seconds hard to 30 seconds moderate

2×1 minute hard to 1 minute moderate

1×2 minute hard to 2 minutes moderate

Repeat steps 2–4

2-minute cool-down

Your Nutrition Tips

If you want to increase lean muscle mass and develop curves, your diet needs to include nutrient and calorie-dense foods and drinks such as seeds, nuts, dried fruits, smoothies, coconut milk, avocados, meats, and protein shakes. In contrast, baked goods, doughnuts, cakes, and fast foods are calorie-dense but not nutrient-dense. Yes, they are tasty, but they are full of empty calories. Even though compared to other body types these type of carbohydrates will not do as much damage to your female ectomorph waistline, you do need to take into consideration your overall health.

When doing workouts in this book, you'll tend to get hungrier between meals, and snacking frequently will allow you to fuel your high metabolism with adequate calories without getting too full from simply eating three enormous meals each day. Although grazing and snacking is not necessarily best for other body types, it can suit your high metabolism quite well. Another very good strategy for consuming adequate calories is to drink your calories by including protein shakes and energy smoothies, preferably from unprocessed natural ingredients with few preservative such as fruit, oil, nuts, milk, and healthy protein powders. Finally, adding toppings to your food is a good way to add healthy extra calories. For example, oils, seeds, nuts, sprouted whole grain, flaxseed crackers, and cubed or crumbled cheese are great additions for both nutrition and flavor.

As mentioned, because of your high metabolism, you can also eat a higher percentage of carbohydrates than the other body types—although these carbohydrates need to ideally come from healthy, nutrient-dense sources such as whole grains, rice, quinoa, amaranth, millet, sweet potatoes, yams, taro, beets, or other natural, minimally processed carbohydrate foods.

If you need help determining exactly how many calories you should eat, please refer to the appendix of this book or to GetFitGuy.com/calculator for a calorie calculator. This will give you a ballpark figure, although you still need to pay attention to your body and hunger levels. You may find that compared to your nonectomorph friends, you need a higher calorie intake to sustain a healthy high metabolism and lean muscle formation.

In fact, you may have trouble actually eating enough food. Usually, this is because ectomorphs tend to be busy, type-A personalities who can get rushed and easily forget to eat, so it can be extremely helpful to log and keep track of your daily food intake. Here are a few other tips to ensure you give yourself enough fuel for curves and lean muscle: try not to eat when you are too stressed or distracted, stop other tasks to eat your meals, and focus on completely chewing each bite of food, even if you're multitasking with a fork in one hand and a smartphone in the other.

If you've increased your calorie intake, are following the

nutrition plan in this book, and still can't seem to gain weight, curves, or muscle, then you may actually have a medical issue. Your physician can determine whether you have hyperthyroidism, one of the more common issues that affect ectomorphs who struggle to gain weight despite high calorie intake.

Sample Daily Meal Plan for Female Ectomorph

Breakfast   HOT CEREAL ▶ ½ cup cooked oatmeal or quinoa with 1 tablespoon of full fat Greek yogurt, 1 teaspoon almond butter, and 1 handful blueberries or 1 banana. Serve with ½ cup almond milk or rice milk.

Morning Snack   1 piece fresh fruit (e.g., a grapefruit or an apple).

Lunch   WHOLE GRAIN TURKEY AVOCADO SANDWICH OR WRAP ▶ 2 slices of whole grain bread or sprouted, gluten-free bread (or wrap), 3–4 slices preservative-free, sodium-free deli turkey, 1 small avocado, ½ tomato, and 1 large handful dark leafy greens like spinach or kale.

or

MIXED BEAN SALAD ▶ Over a handful of lettuce or mixed greens, add ½ diced apple (soaked in lemon juice), 1 tablespoon kidney beans, 1 tablespoon black beans, 1 tablespoon white beans, 1 sliced shallot, and a handful of sliced bell pepper. Dressing is 1 tablespoon red wine vinegar, 1 tablespoon olive oil, 1 teaspoon coconut milk, 1 crushed garlic clove, and 1 teaspoon fresh thyme.

Afternoon Snack   Hummus with fresh vegetables.

Dinner   SALMON PATTIES ON SALAD WITH SWEET POTATOES ▶ Mix 2 cans of wild salmon with ½ cup oats, ½ cup ricotta cheese, 2 eggs,

2 tablespoons each of chopped chives, dill, and cilantro, then a pinch of sea salt and black pepper. Shape into cakes, then add coconut or olive oil to a pan, and lightly fry until golden. Serve with a diced tomato, cucumber, and red onion salad dressed with the same dressing as the mixed bean salad above, and also include sweet potato fries: peel and dice 2 sweet potatoes, coat with olive oil, add a teaspoon each of cumin, turmeric, cinnamon, and sea salt, and bake at 350°F. in a roasting pan for 40 minutes.

Additional Snack Option   1 container full fat Greek yogurt with 10–15 almonds, a handful of blueberries, and ½ dark chocolate bar cut into pieces.

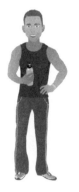

CHAPTER 5

Body Type: Female Mesomorph

I f there is one body type that is a true example of a morph, then it is the mesomorph. This is a commonly seen occurrence in female ex-athletes—several years spent as a trim, fit athlete, followed by a quick morph into a body with excess flab as soon as all that physical activity ceases.

As a female mesomorph, you tend to have a classic hourglass shape, with wide shoulders and hips and a distinctively narrow waist. Because of this shape, you gain and lose weight proportionally in the hips and buttocks, upper back, and chest. Often, because of this even body fat distribution, you can go a long period of time without paying attention to exercise and diet, and then realize one day while looking in the mirror that you've gained a lot of weight!

Fortunately, your mesomorph metabolism (while not fast like that of an ectomorph) is very efficient, and losing fat can seem

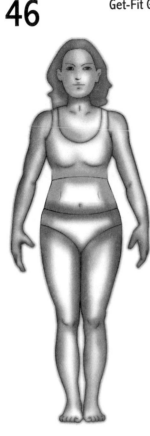

nearly effortless—especially since your body responds very quickly to exercise. At the same time, you need to be careful, since you can gain weight just as easily as you can lose it, and this can lead to frustrating yo-yo fluctuations in your body shape.

The female mesomorph is a natural athlete. You were probably picked first to be on a sports team at school. Because of your naturally high amount of lean muscle, your thicker bones, and your V-shaped torso, you can be good at a variety of sports and activities. Most of the world's top tennis players, soccer players, and bodybuilders are mesomorphs, but this body type is not limited to female athletes such as Serena Williams and Mia Hamm. Many popular female celebrities and entertainers also have mesomorphic body shapes, including Jessica Simpson, Beyoncé Knowles, Scarlett Johansson, Britney Spears, and Jennifer Garner.

Your Strengths

Female mesomorphs might be the most genetically gifted of the body types. With a naturally low body-fat percentage, you tend to be lean, muscular, and athletic without the same amount of effort required by other body types. Another part of your movement superiority is pure physics—a relatively strong upper body and legs combined with a narrow waist can twist, turn, jump, and move with a higher degree of speed and stability.

Wide shoulders and hips combined with a narrow waist also gives you the classic hourglass figure that other body types may envy—which means you may actually be excited when swimsuit season rolls around. A wide variety of clothing fits you well, and even when you gain weight, you don't need to change your entire wardrobe as much as you need to go up in size.

Since you can gain muscle so easily, changing your body shape, becoming more toned, or firming up a trouble spot is not an enormous challenge if you're doing the right workout. You certainly put the "morph" in mesomorph! Your body responds very quickly to physical activity, and when you get into shape, you can have curvaceous and toned buttocks, thighs, arms, and calves.

Your Limitations

Although you are good at quickly gaining muscle and toning your body, this doesn't mean you are bulletproof to fat loss. Since you tend to distribute weight gain evenly throughout your body, you can quickly go up several clothing sizes if you aren't careful about what you eat and how active you style. As mentioned, you often see this pattern in female mesomorph athletes who switch from being highly active to being more sedentary—they suddenly balloon up.

Since this quick weight gain and body fat is evenly distributed, that hourglass waist you have is very prone to deposits of fat above the hip and below the waist. This can be frustrating for you when these muffin tops on your hourglass figure don't allow you to confidently wear jeans and a T-shirt.

In addition, if you are doing the wrong workout program and choosing sets, reps, or weights incorrectly, you can begin to form square, manly shoulders, a thick neck, and a Herculean butt—traits you may not actually desire unless you're a female bodybuilder or you're trying to get a job as a bouncer at your local bar.

Your Ideal Body

If you are engaged in a well-balanced workout program, your chest and shoulders can be well defined and you will have excellent upper body posture that allows you to sit, stand, and carry yourself with grace and ease. Your waist tapers nicely down from your athletic upper body, you can easily get your stomach tight and flat, and if you desire striations or definition in your abdominal musculature, this can also easily be achieved. Your arms and legs tend to be toned and defined, and as you reduce your body fat, this quality is amplified even more.

Even though you are naturally muscular, your butt and thighs don't need to be big and bulky, but instead, with the right combination of cardio and weights, can be lean and toned, with curvaceous calves. To see examples of well-formed female mesomorph body shapes, you can thumb through the photos of female athletes in *ESPN* or *Sports Illustrated* magazines, go watch a sand volleyball tournament, or check out Jillian Michaels, former celebrity trainer on *The Biggest Loser.*

Your Workout Plan

You may be thinking that since you gain muscle so easily you should focus on cardio in your workout plan. But while a cardio-only strategy will help stave off the formation of body fat, it doesn't do much to sculpt and shape your naturally well-defined muscles. Instead, by combining cardio with the proper amount of weight training, you can go from simply having a low body-fat percentage to having an impressive and trim figure.

When you are weight training, a repetition range of 8 to 12 is the volume that tends to cause hypertrophy, or muscle growth. This is actually the repetition range that you'll want to *stay away from* to avoid bulking up. Instead, your female meso-morph weight training routine should be centered around on higher reps (15–25) with relatively lower weights.

Because you won't be training for hypertrophy, your mus-cles probably won't be completely exhausted after a weight training set, so there is no need to rest for long periods of time between exercises, and you can instead do circuit style train-ing, in which you move from one exercise to the next with minimal rest. Since this type of higher rep weight training with shorter rest periods between sets is more cardiovascularly in-tensive, you can count your weights as bonus cardio and worry about doing cardio only on the off days if you have the desire and time permits.

The exercises that you choose for your workout program should consist primarily of full body, multi-joint movements, combined with single-joint movements for trouble spots or parts of your body that you want to tone. The workout program in this book will include instructions for these extra single-joint "vanity exercises." For example, if you want your calves to be more de-fined, you can do the extra routine for calves, or if you wanted your arms to be more toned, do the extra routine for arms.

As mentioned, since you are naturally athletic, you'll re-spond quickly to cardio and don't need to do much of it. But depending on your current weight and body fat stores, if you completely neglect cardio, you will find that you may not have enough calorie-burning activity in your routine. So if this is the case for you, on the days that you aren't weight training or as a warm-up to your weight training routine, focus on high-intensity cardio intervals with a quick warm-up and cool-down. In the workout below, I've included three such high-intensity cardio interval workouts that you can use as a warm-up for your weight training or can do on the off days from your weight training.

Your weight training plan below has three full body, multi-joint circuits that you should space evenly throughout the week. If time permits, at the end of each circuit choose the extra optional vanity exercises that target your personal trouble spot or area you want to tone. You don't need to do all the vanity exercises (or any of them, for that matter)—just the ones that hit the spots you want to work extra.

For a detailed explanation of sets, reps, tempo, load, and other weight training tips, go to "Definitions" in the Appendix (p. 135). You can print workouts to take to the gym with you at GetFitGuy.com.

△ Female Mesomorph Full Body Workout 1

Exercise	Sets	Reps	Tempo	Load
Warm-up: Complete 3–5 minutes of aerobic exercise such as jogging, cycling, or using an elliptical trainer. Or complete the warm-up program in the Appendix of this book (p. 141).				
Main Set: Complete the following circuit of exercises. Rest 60–90 seconds, then repeat, for 2–5 rounds. Beginners should choose a lower number of rounds, while more advanced exercisers can do the higher number.				
Overhead push presses, **p. 206**	2–5	15–20	fluent	65–70%
Pull-ups or pull-downs, **p. 242**	2–5	15–20	fluent	65–70%
Water-ski rows, **p. 231**	2–5	15–20	fluent	65–70%
Single-arm cable chest presses, **p. 237**	2–5	15–20	fluent	65–70%
Romanian dead lifts, **p. 217**	2–5	15–20	fluent	65–70%
Front plank reaches, **p. 191**	2–5	15–20	fluent	body
Vanity Abs 1: Crunches, **p. 195**	2–5	15–20	fluent	body
Vanity Abs 2: Side plank lateral raises, **p. 215**	2–5	15–20	fluent	65–70%
Vanity Arms 1: Dumbbell curls, **p. 207**	2–5	15–20	fluent	65–70%
Vanity Arms 2: Cable triceps push-downs, **p. 240**	2–5	15–20	fluent	65–70%
Vanity Legs 1: Cable leg kickforwards, **p. 239**	2–5	15–20	fluent	65–70%
Vanity Legs 2: Cable leg kickbacks, **p. 239**	2–5	15–20	fluent	65–70%

Cool-down: Finish with 3–5 minutes of light aerobic activity such as cycling or brisk walking, followed by a full body stretch. Visit Tinyurl.com/benstretch for a full body-stretching protocol.

△ Female Mesomorph Full Body Workout 2

Exercise	Sets	Reps	Tempo	Load
Warm-up: Complete 3–5 minutes of aerobic exercise such as jogging, cycling, or using an elliptical trainer. Or complete the warm-up program in the Appendix of this book (p. 141).				
Main Set: Complete the following circuit of exercises. Rest 60–90 seconds, then repeat, for 2–5 rounds. Beginners should choose a lower number of rounds, while more advanced exercisers can do the higher number.				
Straight–arm cable pull-downs, **p. 232**	2–5	15–20	explosive	65–70%
Walking lunges with twist, **p. 222**	2–5	15–20	fluent	65–70%
Cable rows, **p. 230**	2–5	15–20	fluent	65–70%
Push-ups, **p. 187**	2–5	15–20	fluent	body
Barbell or dumbbell squats, **p. 220**	2–5	15–20	fluent	65–70%
Side plank rotations, **p. 216**	2–5	15–20	fluent	body
Vanity Abs 1: Crunches, **p. 195**	2–5	15–20	fluent	body
Vanity Abs 2: Side plank lateral raises, **p. 215**	2–5	15–20	fluent	65–70%
Vanity Arms 1: Alternating biceps curls, **p. 207**	2–5	15–20	fluent	65–70%
Vanity Arms 2: Cable triceps push-downs, **p. 240**	2–5	15–20	fluent	65–70%
Vanity Legs 1: Cable leg kickforwards, **p. 239**	2–5	15–20	fluent	65–70%
Vanity Legs 2: Cable leg kickbacks, **p. 239**	2–5	15–20	fluent	65–70%

Cool-down: Finish with 3–5 minutes of light aerobic activity such as cycling or brisk walking, followed by a full-body stretch. Visit Tinyurl. com/benstretch for a full body-stretching protocol.

△ Female Mesomorph Full Body Workout 3

EXERCISE	SETS	REPS	TEMPO	LOAD
Warm-up: Complete 3–5 minutes of aerobic exercise such as jogging, cycling, or using an elliptical trainer. Or complete the warm-up program in the Appendix of this book (p. 141).				
Main Set: Complete the following circuit of exercises. Rest 60–90 seconds, then repeat, for 2–5 rounds. Beginners should choose a lower number of rounds, while more advanced exercisers can do the higher number.				
Goblet squats, **p. 212**	2–5	15–20	fluent	65–70%
Ball leg curls, **p. 227**	2–5	15–20	fluent	65–70%
Single-arm dumbbell rows, **p. 209**	2–5	15–20	fluent	65–70%
Incline push-ups, **p. 189**	2–5	15–20	fluent	body
Cable chest flies, **p. 236**	2–5	15–20	fluent	65–70%
Cable torso twists, **p. 230**	2–5	15–20	fluent	65–70%
Vanity Abs 1: Crunches, **p. 195**	2–5	15–20	fluent	body
Vanity Abs 2: Side plank lateral raises, **p. 215**	2–5	15–20	fluent	65–70%
Vanity Arms 1: Dumbbell curls, **p. 207**	2–5	15–20	fluent	65–70%
Vanity Arms 2: Cable triceps push-downs, **p. 240**	2–5	15–20	fluent	65–70%
Vanity Legs 1: Cable leg kickforwards, **p. 239**	2–5	15–20	fluent	65–70%
Vanity Legs 2: Cable leg kickbacks, **p. 239**	2–5	15–20	fluent	65–70%

Cool-down: Finish with 3–5 minutes of light aerobic activity such as cycling or brisk walking, followed by a full-body stretch. Visit Tinyurl.com/benstretch for a full body-stretching protocol.

On the days that you are not weight training or as a warm-up for your weight training workouts, you can perform the following cardio interval workouts on a bicycle, treadmill, elliptical trainer, or rowing machine, or walking or running outdoors. Remember that the minimal rest in your weight training circuits are already giving you significant amounts of cardio, so the workouts below are optional, and need to be included only if you want to accelerate weight loss or significantly improve cardiovascular fitness.

High Intensity Cardio Interval Workout 1

> *5-minute warm-up*
>
> *3 minutes at a hard effort, followed by 1 minute at very high intensity*
>
> *4 minutes at a moderate pace*
>
> *2 minutes at a hard effort, followed by 1 minute at very high intensity*
>
> *3 minutes at a moderate pace*
>
> *1 minute at a hard effort, followed by 1 minute at very high intensity*
>
> *2 minutes at a moderate pace*
>
> *3-minute cool-down*

High Intensity Cardio Interval Workout 2

> *5 minutes at a moderate pace*
>
> *3×30 seconds hard to 30 seconds moderate*
>
> *2×1 minute hard to 1 minute moderate*
>
> *1×2 minute hard to 2 minutes moderate*
>
> *Repeat steps 2–4 one more time*
>
> *2-minute cool-down*

High Intensity Cardio Interval Workout 3

> *5 minutes at a moderate pace*
> *3×30 seconds hard to 30 seconds moderate*
> *2×1 minute hard to 1 minutes moderate*
> *1×2 minute hard to 2 minute moderate*
> *Repeat steps 2–4*
> *2-minute cool-down*

Your Nutrition Tips

As a mesomorph, if you aren't careful with how much you eat, you can easily gain weight quickly and distribute fat everywhere, so your goal should be to prioritize nutrient-dense foods, and include high calorie foods only as strategically timed energy for your workouts.

Although you do not have the sky-high appetite of the female ectomorph, you will still tend to get hungry between meals, so you should be sure to have at least two healthy snacks on hand during the day—one for between breakfast and lunch and another for between lunch and dinner. The first snack of the day should be more carbohydrate rich, since your metabolism will be higher early in the day. As a female, you must consume enough fat to give your body the building blocks for hormones. That's why your afternoon snack should be more fat based and primarily include healthy fats that contain high levels of omega-3 fatty acids (like walnuts), monounsaturated fats (like olives), and medium chain triglycerides (like coconut-based foods). You'll also need fewer carbohydrates, and these should instead be replaced with lean proteins to repair your muscle fibers.

If you need help determining exactly how many calories you should eat, go to GetFitGuy.com/calculator for a calorie calculator. This will give you a ballpark figure, although you still need to pay attention to your body and hunger levels, especially if you are doing all the weight training and the cardio intervals in this chapter.

If you're watching your calorie intake and following the nutrition plan in this book, and find that you seem to still be putting on body fat, you may want to consider filling in any nutritional deficiencies with supplementation. Deficiencies in vitamin D, magnesium, digestive enzymes, and probiotics are common in active or athletic females. Make sure to have your doctor test your levels before starting on any supplement program.

Sample Daily Meal Plan for Female Mesomorph

Breakfast   EGGS AND VEGGIES ▸ Fry or scramble 2 to 3 free-range, omega-3-enriched eggs in coconut oil and add tomato slices, spinach, red onions, ½ an avocado, and a handful of feta or cheddar cheese. Serve with a slice of sprouted whole grain toast, or inside a wrap with salsa.

Morning Snack   1 piece fresh fruit (e.g., a grapefruit or an apple).

Lunch   PROTEIN SALAD ▸ Over a bed of mixed greens, kale, or any other dark leafy green, add ½ an avocado, ½ a can of sardines in olive oil, or 4–6 ounces any other meat of choice, a small handful of feta cheese, 6–8 olives, a sliced tomato, and any other vegetables of choice. Use olive oil and balsamic vinaigrette as dressing, or just use oil from sardines.

Afternoon Snack   Greek yogurt with handful of almonds.

Dinner   VEGETABLE PILAF WITH FISH ▶ Heat for about 10 minutes in a lightly oiled or buttered saucepan 2 chopped onions, 2 cloves garlic, 2 tablespoons ginger, 1 teaspoon ground cinnamon, and 2 whole cloves (spice to taste). Add 1–2 cups of wild or brown rice. Add 1–2 cups of peas. Add 3 cups of vegetable stock or water. Simmer until rice is cooked. Serve with 4–6 ounces salmon, halibut, cod, or other fish, prepared as desired. Refrigerate leftover plate.

CHAPTER 6

Body Type:
Female Endo-Mesomorph

If you've ever seen female nudes in paintings from the Renaissance, then you've probably seen your body type. Today commonly referred to as the pear, people of your shape usually have wide hips, buttocks, and thighs combined with narrow shoulders and a thin waist. Your weight gain tends to accumulate more in your upper legs and thighs than in your upper body or lower legs.

I personally am not a fan of the term *pear* because it makes it sound as though you have a fat and flabby lower body combined with a tiny, weak upper body—and this definitely does not need to be the case! Although it is true that an out-of-shape female meso-endomorph can have a frail upper body with a disproportionately larger lower half, with the proper workout program you can easily balance your dimensions. One female meso-endomorph who successfully achieved this (Jennifer

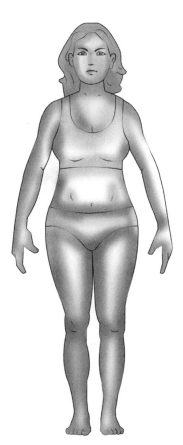

Lopez) was named *People* magazine's most beautiful woman in 2011!

Your upper body is proportionally smaller and you may have a hard time adding muscle, tone, or definition to this area. Instead, you easily put on both excess weight and added muscle in your lower body—particularly the hips, butt, and thighs. This is because your body naturally distributes fat in these areas first. But if your body-fat percentage increases significantly, you may find that you also can gain extra weight in your waist and upper stomach.

Your shoulders are narrower than or similar in width to your hips. Even if you are out of shape or overweight, you waist appears to be relatively narrow, especially compared with your lower half, and your bust measurement is smaller than your hip measurement. Although calf sizes vary among female endo-mesomorphs, you easily add muscle and tone to your calves.

Examples of celebrity meso-endomorphs also include Minnie Driver, Kim Kardashian, Anna Kournikova, and Halle Berry. Each of these women, as well as many other actresses and singers (especially African-American and Latina women), are perfect examples of how beautiful and curvaceous the female meso-endomorph body can be with the proper workout and nutrition program.

Your Strengths

You really don't have to worry much about weight gain in your upper body, since it is relatively easy for you to tone your shoulders, chest, and arms. This, combined with your naturally narrow waist, means that you don't have to work hard to have a fit upper body and can instead do just a few strategic workouts to get quick results for this section.

Because your hips, butt, and thighs are so shapely, the right workout program can give you an incredible pair of legs, and you can look fantastic in shorts, skirts, and jeans. If you are in shape, your lower body can also be great for sports that require short explosive movements such as the sprinting, jumping, and landing required for basketball or track. With the proper toning and strengthening program for your arms, chest, and shoulders, you can make sure your upper and lower body are in the proper proportion to each other—and you can have a classically beautiful female figure.

Your Limitations

As you probably already know, if you don't watch what you eat and maintain the right exercise program, you can easily put on weight. Your metabolism is slower than that of a female ectomorph or mesomorph, and a combination of calorie control and choosing the right foods is essential for you to attain your dream body.

Your upper body can be weak and unbalanced, which not only affects the overall aesthetic balance of your body and the way your clothes fit but can also give you a propensity for shoulder or arm injuries.

Since your hips tend to be wider, you may have some difficulty with hip, knee, ankle, or foot injuries when you do repetitive-motion activities such as running or bicycling. This can be addressed by putting orthotics in your shoes and getting a proper bike fit, but can be frustrating if you're interested in these activities.

Your Ideal Body

You can slim out your hips, thighs, and buttocks, achieve a killer pair of legs, and balance your upper body with a tight and toned chest, shoulders, and arms. This allows your natural pear shape to be well proportioned and symmetrical. Your shoulders, chest, and arms, when firm and defined, complement your naturally narrow waist. As you lower the percentage of body fat in your upper legs and add definition to your naturally lean and muscular calves, you can achieve a shapely, trim, and athletic lower body.

Many well-known endo-mesomorph celebrities have achieved this dream body, including Jennifer Lopez, Beyoncé Knowles, Kim Kardashian, Eva Longoria, and Shakira. Looking at images of these women will give you an idea of the shape you can achieve.

Your Workout Plan

Your exercise program needs to take into account the difference in strength, functionality, and appearance between your upper body and your lower body. For this reason, the workout program for your arms, chest and shoulders needs to prioritize the production of force and lean muscle development, with medium to heavy weights and multi-joint movements. In contrast, your lower body workouts should include only a small amount of light to medium weight training. Your leg exercise should focus on high intensity interval cardio to boost your metabolism and aerobic, steady cardio to burn fat.

The best way to structure such a workout program will be to focus on high quality isolation of body sections by separating your upper body weight training workouts from your lower body cardio and weights days. For example, you can do an upper body workout two to three days per week, then do cardio (such as running or bicycling) and a lower body workout on another two to three days of the week.

For strength, lean muscle development, and a balanced look, your upper body weight training range should be around 8–10 repetitions of a weight that you find challenging, while your lower body weight training range can be 15–20 repetitions with lighter weights. By doing your lower body weight training immediately before or after your cardio sessions, you can accelerate the rate of fat loss and toning in the hips, butt, and thighs.

For the workout program below, do the upper body circuit two to three days per week. Do the lower body on a different two to three days, preferably either before or after the cardio session for that day. If you're highly motivated or in shape, then exercise on more days per week.

Finally, you'll notice that there are alternative movements to each of the exercises. Since you should ideally be switching up your workouts every four to six weeks, these will come in handy. To see examples of alternative pushing, pulling, rowing, twisting, extending, and other exercises, simply visit GetFitGuy .com/exercises.

For a detailed explanation of sets, reps, tempo, load, and other weight training tips, go to "Definitions" in the Appendix (p. 135). You can print workouts to take to the gym with you at GetFitGuy.com.

△ *Female Endo-Mesomorph Upper Body Workout*

EXERCISE	SETS	REPS	TEMPO	LOAD
Warm-up: Complete 3-5 minutes of aerobic exercise such as jogging, cycling, or using an elliptical trainer. Or complete the warm-up program in the Appendix of this book (p. 141).				
Main Set: Complete the following circuit of exercises. Rest 60–90 seconds, then repeat, for 2–5 rounds. Beginners should choose a lower number of rounds, while more advanced exercisers can do the higher number.				
Cable chest press, **p. 236**	2–4	8–10	fluent	80–85%
Dumbbell overhead press, **p. 205**	2–4	8–10	fluent	80–85%
Pull-downs, **p. 232**	2–4	8–10	fluent	80–85%
Single-arm dumbbell rows, **p. 209**	2–4	8–10	fluent	80–85%
Cable torso twists, **p. 230**	2–4	8–10	fluent	80–85%
Front plank reaches, **p. 191**	2–4	8–10	fluent	body

Cool-down: Finish with 3–5 minutes of light aerobic activity such as cycling or brisk walking, followed by a full body stretch. Visit Tinyurl.com/benstretch for a full body-stretching protocol.

△ Female Endo-Mesomorph Lower Body Workout with Cardio

EXERCISE	SETS	REPS	TEMPO	LOAD
Warm-up: Complete 3–5 minutes of aerobic exercise such as jogging, cycling or using an elliptical trainer. Or complete the warm-up program in the Appendix of this book (p. 141).				
Main Set: Complete the following circuit of exercises. Rest 60–90 seconds, then repeat, for 2–5 rounds. Beginners should choose a lower number of rounds, while more advanced exercisers can do the higher number.				
Squats, **p. 197**	3–5	20–25	fluent	body
Lateral lunges, **p. 198**	3–5	20–25	fluent	body
Ball leg curls, **p. 227**	3–5	20–25	fluent	body
Cable abduction, **p. 238**	3–5	20–25	fluent	60–65%
Cable adduction, **p. 238**	3–5	20–25	fluent	60–65%
Kickouts, **p. 192**	3–5	20–25	fluent	body
Ball knee-ups, **p. 225**	3–5	10–15	fluent	body

Cool-down: Finish with 3–5 minutes of light aerobic activity such as cycling or brisk walking, followed by a full body stretch. Visit Tinyurl.com/benstretch for a full body-stretching protocol.

Additional Instructions: Include one of the following either before or after your workout:

1. 20–45 minutes running, cycling, elliptical or other leg aerobic cardio at a steady, moderate pace.
2. Using running, cycling, elliptical or other leg cardio, perform 5-minute warm-up, then 2 minutes very hard followed by 1 minute easy, 5–10 times through.

Your Nutrition Tips

To avoid feeling chronically fatigued and stressed, as an endo-mesomorph, you will need additional calories and nutrients to support the workout program above. But because your metabolism tends to be slower and you gain weight in response to foods with higher sugar content, you should be sure to strategize when you eat in relation to when you exercise (especially when it comes to carbohydrates).

You'll be able to trim and tone your lower body more quickly and effectively if you perform your lower body workouts and cardio in the morning, prior to breakfast. If that isn't possible, try to do them in the late afternoon or evening without having had an afternoon snack. This may be tough for the first few days as you learn to tap into your own storage fat, but you'll eventually adapt.

Your overall caloric intake should be skewed toward natural proteins like fish and healthy fats like seeds and nuts, with fewer carbohydrates or energy-dense foods. In addition, you should try as much as possible to use the strategy of carbohydrate timing, which means that breakfast and your first snack of the day should be more carbohydrate rich, since your metabolism will be higher early in the day—and your afternoon snack should include more fats and proteins. For example, your morning snack can be a piece of fresh fruit, and your afternoon snack could be a handful of olives or walnuts, or sliced avocado with sea salt.

If you need help determining exactly how many calories you should eat, go to GetFitGuy.com/calculator for a calorie calculator. This will give you a ballpark figure, although you still need to pay attention to your body and hunger levels, especially if you are doing all the weight training and cardio intervals in this chapter.

If you're watching your calorie intake, following the nutrition plan in this book, and find that you seem to still be putting on body fat, you may want to consider whether you have any hormonal deficiencies or imbalances. An endocrinologist, registered dietitian, or nutritional therapist can help you test, identify, and treat any issues (such as estrogen dominance) that may be hindering your progress.

Sample Daily Meal Plan for Female Endo-Mesomorph

Breakfast YOGURT PARFAIT ▸ One small container of plain full-fat yogurt with a handful of blueberries or raspberries and a handful of almonds, walnuts, or macadamia nuts or a tablespoon of nut butter.

Morning Snack 1 piece fresh and fruit (e.g., a grapefruit or an apple).

Lunch PROTEIN SALAD ▸ Over a bed of mixed greens, kale, or any other dark leafy green, add ½ an avocado, ½ a can of sardines in olive oil, or 4–6 ounces any other meat of choice, a small handful of feta cheese, 6–8 olives, a sliced tomato, and any other vegetables of choice. Use olive oil and balsamic vinaigrette as dressing, or just use the oil from the sardines.

Afternoon Snack Eat a small- to medium-sized avocado, sliced, with a few pieces of cheese of your choice and salt and pepper to taste.

Dinner CHICKEN SKEWERS WITH ALMOND SAUCE ▸ Cut chicken breasts into ½-inch cubes. Marinate in low-sodium soy or low-sugar teriyaki sauce for about 2 hours. Barbecue chicken on skewer or bake at 350°F. until cooked through. Place on a big bed of spinach and serve with almond sauce.

For almond sauce, in a saucepan over medium heat, combine 1 tablespoon almond butter, 2 teaspoons honey, 2 teaspoons soy or teriyaki sauce, 1 tablespoon brown rice vinegar, 2 teaspoons grated ginger, and ½ cup coconut milk. Cook until sauce thickens, or about 5 minutes.

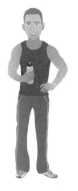

CHAPTER 7

Body Type:
Female Endomorph

I f the female meso-endomorph is a pear, then you are the other body shape fruit: the apple. As a female endomorph, you are slightly smaller on the top half of your body than on the bottom half. You tend to have wider hips and smaller shoulders, a medium to large bust, thick joints and large bones, shorter arms and legs, with thick wrists and ankles. Your body fat is not evenly distributed across your whole body, being primarily located on your lower stomach, butt, hips, and thighs, which contributes to your curvaceous, round shape. Celebrity female endomorphs include Queen Latifah, Oprah Winfrey, Jennifer Coolidge, and Kate Winslet.

Because you burn fat very efficiently, you are better at long, slow cardiovascular exercise, such as jogging or cycling. Although you can gain muscle easily, you are not naturally strong or powerful, and do better moving light weights for

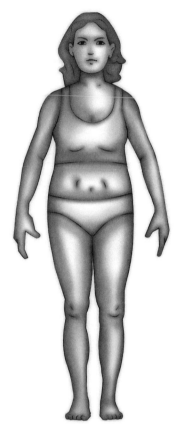

more repetitions or for longer periods of time. The key to weight loss for you is tapping into your storage body fat levels with consistent physical activity while maintaining as much lean muscle as possible. But this can't be achieved simply through nutrition, which is why exercise and movement is crucial for female endomorphs.

Your body is soft, curvy, and round primarily because of your natural bone structure, your higher percentage of body fat, and a slower metabolism. While this means you can gain weight easily and have to work hard to lose body fat, it also means that you have womanly curves—and that's why some of the sexiest celebrity singers and actresses, such as Janet Jackson and Britney Spears are endomorphs!

Your Strengths

You have impressive curves that make other women jealous. When you do the proper combination of cardio and weights, you don't lose your curves or your shape as some other female body types do, but instead add tone and definition to your physique, allowing you to achieve a sexy look. The female endomorph body can be voluptuous, alluring, and sensual— think of Sophia Loren or Kate Winslet.

Because cardiovascular exercise uses a higher percentage of fat as fuel, you naturally excel at covering long distances. As an Ironman triathlete, I see many endomorphs do very well at such races after they've lost weight, because of that natural cardiovascular talent.

Your Limitations

Because of your sluggish metabolism, you will have a harder time losing weight compared to other body types. Your naturally higher body fat percentage means that you may need to exercise for longer periods of time before you begin to actually see muscle tone and definition. That doesn't mean it is impossible for you to get your dream body—it just means that you need to be consistent with both exercise and nutrition planning and execution. You can gain fat very quickly if you eat the wrong types of foods or just slightly more than you actually need, so it can be tough for you to lose weight through diet alone. Exercise is essential for you to get your dream body.

Because you're better at cardiovascular exercise, strong and powerful efforts can be difficult for you, as can short sprinting or fast running. If you're overweight, even moderate cardiovascular exercise can feel harder than it should, although you will find that as you shed pounds or lower your body fat percentage, cardio becomes easier.

Finally, cellulite tends to be an issue for female endomorphs and endo-mesomorphs. So if you're seeing cottage cheese–like fat deposits on your buttocks, thighs, or upper legs (the most common areas), then you should head over GetFitGuy.Quick andDirtyTips.com and read the two-part article series "What Causes Cellulite" and "How to Get Rid of Cellulite."

Your Ideal Body

As an endomorph, you can look absolutely amazing. When you're in shape, your soft, curvaceous look is balanced with toned and fit arms and legs, an inward curve of the waist, and a large, round bust. This womanly shape cannot be achieved by any other body type, and no matter how hard she tries, a female ectomorph can never equal your curves.

Of course, at the same time, you should realize that because of your naturally higher percentage of body fat and lean muscle, you will never achieve the low body fat percentage and narrow shape of an ectomorph. The key to achieving *your* ideal body is to burn the storage fat that tends to settle in the curvaceous lower regions (such as your lower abdomen, butt, hips, and thighs) while toning and strengthening your relatively smaller shoulders and upper body. When this is achieved, your apple shape becomes compact while still maintaining voluptuous curves. Your shoulders, chest, and arms will be tight and toned; your stomach will be flat, but with a natural softness. Your hips, butt, and thighs will be curvaceous but not flabby, and your lower legs, like your upper body, will have a tight and toned look.

Your Workout Plan

Since you burn fewer calories than other types, your entire workout program should be structured around consistent cardiovascular exercise, with small amounts of weight training used for extra toning. Single-joint exercises such as biceps curls and triceps extensions, or spot-reducing exercises such as crunches, don't burn many calories and are extremely in-effective for the endomorph body type. Instead, most of your exercises should use multiple body parts, which will boost your metabolism and burn more calories.

Exercise consistency is key for your metabolic rate, and rather than simply doing a few significantly long cardio sessions a couple of days per week, you should instead try to perform shorter cardio sessions on as many days of the week as you can. Whenever possible, you should do your cardio on an empty stomach, in a fasted state, such as immediately in the morning prior to breakfast. Fortunately, you don't have to worry about getting light-headed or running out of energy, since for these sessions you'll be exercising in a zone that targets storage fat as the primary energy source. High intensity cardiovascular intervals, which are harder on your joints and body and use more carbohydrate as fuel, should not be a significant part of your exercise routine.

If you are overweight, then the activity you choose for cardiovascular exercise should be easy on your hips, knees, and ankles. So instead of pounding away miles on the treadmill, better choices for you are using the elliptical trainer, cycling, hiking, power walking, water aerobics, and swimming. Because your body adapts quickly to the demands you place on it, you should switch up your cardio modes as often as possible.

For weight training, you should be doing a short, full body exercise circuit two to three times per week, with minimal rest between sets, 12–15 repetitions per set and 2–4 sets per exercise. You can do these on the same day as your cardio sessions (preferably at a different time of the day), or on the days in between your cardio sessions. You should also change up your weight training exercises at least once every four weeks.

As your cardio burns fat, your weight training will be causing slight increases in muscle. Since muscle weighs more than fat, you may find yourself better motivated by tracking your decrease in body fat percentage instead of your decrease in weight, since your weight may not lower significantly fast.

Below you will find two female endomorph workouts that include a full body exercise circuit for weight training, along with short cardio bursts. In addition, you'll find intensity recommendations and instructions for your longer, slower cardio sessions.

Besides performing the workouts below, you may find it beneficial for you to make adjustments in your day-to-day routine, such as standing as much as possible, taking the stairs, or parking farther from the door of stores. Check out GetFitGuy.QuickandDirtyTips.com for a great article on "7 Ways to Burn Calories by Standing More."

For a detailed explanation of sets, reps, tempo, load, and other weight training tips, go to "Definitions" in the Appendix (p. 135). You can print workouts to take to the gym with you at GetFitGuy.com.

△ *Female Endomorph Full Body Workout 1*

EXERCISE	SETS	REPS	TEMPO	LOAD
Warm-up: Complete 3–5 minutes of aerobic exercise such as jogging, cycling, or using an elliptical trainer. Or complete the warm-up program in the Appendix of this book (p. 141).				
Main Set: Complete the following circuit of exercises. Rest 60–90 seconds, then repeat, for 2–4 rounds. Beginners should choose a lower number of rounds, while more advanced exercisers can do the higher number. IMPORTANT: Finish each circuit with 30–60 seconds of intense cardio (e.g., elliptical or cycling).				
Cable chest press, **p. 236**	2–4	12–15	fluent	70–75%
Cable seated row, **p. 234**	2–4	12–15	fluent	70–75%
Dumbbell overhead press, **p. 205**	2–4	12–15	fluent	70–75%
Cable pull-downs, **p. 232**	2–4	12–15	fluent	70–75%
Ball bridges, **p. 226**	2–4	12–15	fluent	body
Machine leg extensions*	2–4	12–15	fluent	70–75%
Machine leg curls*	2–4	12–15	fluent	70–75%
Machine leg press*	2–4	12–15	fluent	70–75%
Cool-down: Finish with 3–5 minutes of light aerobic activity such as cycling or brisk walking, followed by a full body stretch. Visit Tinyurl.com/benstretch for a full body-stretching protocol.				

*For these, and many other exercises, go to GetFitGuy.com.

△ *Female Endomorph Full Body Workout 2*

EXERCISE	SETS	REPS	TEMPO	LOAD
Warm-Up: Complete 3–5 minutes of aerobic exercise such as jogging, cycling, or using an elliptical trainer. Or complete the warm-up program in the Appendix of this book (p. 141).				
Main Set: Complete the following circuit of exercises. Rest 60–90 seconds, then repeat, for 2–4 rounds. Beginners should choose a lower number of rounds, while more advanced exercisers can do the higher number. IMPORTANT: Finish each circuit with 30–60 seconds of intense cardio (e.g., elliptical or cycling).				
Goblet squats, **p. 212**	2–4	12–15	fluent	70–75%
Walking lunges, **p. 213**	2–4	12–15	fluent	70–75%
Cable torso twists, **p. 230**	2–4	12–15	fluent	70–75%
Dumbbell chest presses, **p. 228**	2–4	12–15	fluent	70–75%
Pull-ups or pull-downs, **p. 242**	2–4	12–15	fluent	70–75%
Dumbbell shoulder presses, **p. 205**	2–4	12–15	fluent	70–75%
Dumbbell rows, **p. 209**	2–4	12–15	fluent	70–75%

Cool-down: Finish with 3–5 minutes of light aerobic activity such as cycling or brisk walking, followed by a full body stretch. Visit Tinyurl.com/benstretch for a full body-stretching protocol.

In addition to the workouts above, you should perform 30–60 minutes of fat-burning cardio on as many days of the week as possible, preferably in the morning prior to breakfast. Because these sessions are at a slower rate and can be as simple as a brisk walk out your front door, you don't need to worry that you will overtrain your body by doing them every day. Ideally, you should purchase a heart rate monitor to make sure that you perform these sessions in your maximum fat-burning heart rate zone.

Once you have a heart rate monitor, here are instructions for finding your personalized fat-burning zone more accurately:

- Warm up on a bike for 10 minutes.
- Pedal at your maximum sustainable pace for 20 minutes. You should be breathing hard and your legs should be burning, but you should be able to maintain the same intensity for the full 20 minutes.
- Record your average heart rate during those 20 minutes.
- Subtract 20 beats from that heart rate. Add and subtract 3 beats from the resulting number to get a range. That is your peak fat-burning zone.

Here's an example. Let's say your average heart rate was 160 during the 20-minute pedal session: $160 - 20 = 140$. Then $140 + 3 = 143$, $140 - 3 = 137$. So your peak fat-burning zone is when you have a heart rate of 137 to 143 beats per minute.

Compared with the results I have obtained from hundreds of individuals in a professional exercise physiology lab with all sorts of gas masks and gadgets, this method obtains accurate fat-burning zone results. But if you did want to have a laboratory test. to find your personal fat-burning zone, then you should look for something called an exercise metabolic rate test, also known as a VO_2 max test.

Your Nutrition Tips

The most important concept for you to understand is that since your body fat percentage is naturally higher, your body can very easily rely on its own fat stores as a steady supply of energy. But there are several things that can keep this from happening, including a very low calorie diet, which can suppress metabolic rate and fat burning; constantly snacking, especially on carbohydrate-rich foods, which can keep your body clinging to its fat reserves; and eating too many pre- and post-workout meals. In other words, don't starve yourself, ignore the advice you hear to snack all the time, and don't go overboard with the fancy pre- and post-exercise shakes and bars.

You will tend to be highly sensitive to carbohydrate intake, so you should eat lots of lower calorie, nutrient-dense vegetables and lean protein, moderate amounts of healthy fats, and a few strategically timed carbohydrates. Seemingly healthy foods that may not cause weight gain for other body types, such as sweet potatoes or yams, can still be a problem for you, which is why your ectomorphic friend's diet just won't work for you.

If you need help determining exactly how many calories you should eat, go to GetFitGuy.com/calculator for a calorie calculator. This will give you a ballpark figure, although you still need to pay attention to your body and your hunger levels, especially if you are doing all the weight training and cardio intervals in this program.

Female endomorphs naturally feel more tired and fatigued, especially if they are overdoing exercise, so try not to go significantly above the recommendations you find in this book. If you're watching your calorie intake, following the nutrition plan, and still putting on body fat, you may want to consider whether you have any hormonal deficiencies or imbalances. An endocrinologist, registered dietitian, or nutritional therapist can help you test, identify, and treat any issues (such as estrogen dominance) that may be hindering your progress.

Sample Daily Meal Plan for Female Endomorph

Breakfast   BREAKFAST SCRAMBLE ▸ Scramble 2–3 eggs with a small handful of cheddar cheese, a handful of spinach, 1 diced tomato, 1 large sliced avocado and garlic, and add salt and pepper to taste.

Lunch   PROTEIN SALAD ▸ Over a bed of mixed greens, kale, or any other dark leafy green, add half an avocado, half a can of sardines in olive oil, or 4–6 ounces of any other meat of choice, a small handful of feta cheese, 6–8 olives, a sliced tomato, and any other vegetables of choice. Use olive oil and balsamic vinaigrette as dressing, or just use the oil from the sardines.

Pre- or Post-Workout Snack (before or after weight training sessions only) 1 piece of fresh fruit with a handful of raw almonds or walnuts.

Dinner   BAKED FISH WITH VEGETABLES ▸ Place a fillet of fish (4–6 ounces) on a large piece of foil. Add ½ cup sliced carrots and ½ cup sliced zucchini, and sprinkle fish and vegetables with lemon juice, parsley, lemon- pepper, sea salt, and dill. Fold foil over and fold edges in twice, forming a pouch. Place on a baking sheet and bake at 450°F. for 15–20 minutes, or until the vegetables are tender and the fish is flaking.

Alternatively, if you're not a fish fan, just bake the vegetables and serve with chicken or steak prepared as desired!

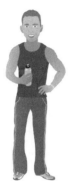

CHAPTER 8

Body Type: Male Ectomorph

If you flip through men's fitness or health magazines or visit a typical bodybuilding or weight lifting Web site, one phrase is consistently used to describe the male ectomorph body type: hard-gainer. Your body is described as a hard-gainer because of the tough time you experience trying to gain any significant amount of muscle. This may not be a big deal to you because you happen to be good at sports involving physical endurance, such as running and cycling—but if you do want to pack on muscle or get bigger, this hard-gainer business can be quite frustrating.

With skinny arms, wrists, legs, ankles, and a thin waist, you have a very linear, stick shape, and when you do gain weight, it tends to go to the front of your stomach and the sides of your waist, just above your hips (the classic beer belly). The good news is that with the proper workout program, you can use

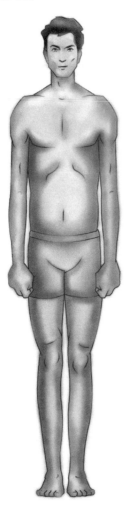

your naturally lean look to your advantage. If you flip through the first few pages of *GQ* magazine, you'll see many ectomorphic male models who have managed to add just enough muscle to make their skinny body look great. Celebrity examples of male ectomorphs include Lance Armstrong, Clint Eastwood, Ethan Hawke, Billy Bob Thornton, Michael Cera, and Chris Rock.

Your Strengths

If a female ectomorph has the high metabolism of a speeding sports car, you as a male ectomorph have the screamingly high metabolism of a fighter jet. This is because ectomorphs have a naturally elevated metabolic rate, and compared with your female counterparts, you male ectomorphs have even higher amounts of metabolism-boosting lean muscle fibers. So what does this mean for you?

First, you can eat enormous amounts of food without gaining significant weight. Think of your metabolism as a garbage disposal—able to process huge amounts of calories, whether those calories are junk food or healthy fare. Of course indiscriminate consumption of whatever you want to eat has consequences for your health, but this excess food certainly has a much harder time sticking to your waistline.

Second, your type of metabolism and muscle fiber is good at long bouts of physical endurance, and you can exercise at low intensities for long periods of time without stopping or getting tired. For this reason, the Tour de

France is probably one of the only sports events in the world comprised purely of ectomorphs.

Finally, because your body fat is naturally low, muscle that is added from a proper exercise program will be well defined and easy to notice. The trick is to learn how to actually add the muscle!

Your Limitations

Sports that require large amounts of power and strength may be difficult or intimidating for you, and heavy lifting, pushing, pulling, sprinting, or high impact activities can leave you sore and beat up. But you need to include activities that require explosiveness or lifting heavier amounts of weight, since this is the only way to keep your small frame, bones, and muscles strong.

Indeed, even if it is not your goal to get big, gain muscle mass, or have more muscularly defined arms and legs, you are liable to get injured and to have poor posture and low hormones due to lack of muscle. In other words, you need hit the weights for more reason than simply "working on your guns," and you need to weight train if you want to keep your body functioning well for life.

On the other hand, if becoming more muscular actually is your goal, then because of your muscle fiber composition, high metabolism, and smaller frame, you will need to work significantly harder at that goal than the other male body types. For a male ectomorph, gaining muscle is just not as simple as waltzing into the gym for the occasional casual weight training routine.

Because of your high metabolism, you may also find that you need to eat annoyingly large amounts of calories if you want to gain size. Before you rush off to grab a Big Mac and fries, bear in mind that these calories need to come from nutrient-dense foods, not fast foods or processed, packaged "frankenfoods." Here's where your high metabolism can be a disadvantage. Cell-damaging free radicals, wrinkles, and even a shortened life span can result from a combination of a high metabolism and a high calorie diet of unhealthy foods. Think of it like having your car's engine revved all the time while you dump dirty gasoline into the tank—it simply won't last quite as long.

Your Ideal Body

As mentioned earlier, many male models are ectomorphs on whose long and lean bodies most clothing fits well. In addition, if you've added a little bit of muscle to your skinny arms and legs, you can look good with your shirt off too, especially since your body fat is so naturally low.

While you'll never have the Herculean look of a barrel chest, bulging biceps, thick, muscular thighs, and large, square calves, with the right workout program you can achieve a body that looks like Brad Pitt in the movie *Fight Club* or Tobey Maguire in *Spider Man*. Not bad!

Your relatively small shoulders and chest can be tight and striated with lean muscle, while your arms can have lean but defined biceps and triceps. If you do too much cardiovascular exercise, your legs can look skinny and stringy, like those of a marathon runner, but with a combination of heavier weight training and a small amount of high intensity interval training, you can instead have legs that look more like Lance Armstrong's— muscular thighs and impressive calves.

Although your stomach and outside of your waistline are definitely the first places you tend to deposit fat, it will not be hard for you to have a flat, hard stomach if you make a few dietary adjustments. To see examples of impressive male ectomorph body types, do an Internet search for images of Brad Pitt, Lance Armstrong, and Clint Eastwood in his younger days, or just thumb through the first several pages of men's fashion and pop culture magazines.

Your Workout Plan

Brace yourself, because to get your ideal body, you may need to make a drastic adjustment to your current exercise routine. As a male ectomorph, you have a high number of slow twitch muscle fibers, which produce low amounts of force and appear small and skinny. In contrast, fast twitch muscle can produce the muscular, filled-out look that can make your skinny body look more impressive (although Olympic gold medal sprinter Usain Bolt is actually an ecto-mesomorph, he is a perfect example of a what a skinny guy can look like with more fast twitch muscle fiber).

Although some slow twitch muscle fibers can be converted to fast twitch muscle fibers, you should focus on adding extra fast twitch muscle fibers to your body by engaging in a full body power and strength weight training program. By simultaneously avoiding high amounts of aerobic exercise, you can then ensure that those precious fast twitch muscles do not atrophy or decrease in size. Whether your goal is to get big or simply to look better with your shirt off, fast twitch muscle fibers will allow you to achieve that goal. The amount you actually eat and lift will affect how much muscle you actually add.

In most cases, male ectomorphs do not lift a heavy enough weight to stimulate their hard-gainer body to put on much muscle at all. While high-repetition, low-weight sets of 12, 15, or 20 reps will work for the other male body types, such sets are simply a waste of time for you, and primarily serve to stimulate your slow twitch muscle fibers. As a personal trainer, I typically find that my skinny guy clients are shocked when they realize how much weight they actually need to lift to see size or definition results.

When you switch to a heavier weight training program that can add muscle definition, most of your exercises should be done with free weights such as barbells or dumbbells, since these will allow you to lift heavier weights than you can with other common exercise tools such as elastic bands, cables, medicine balls, or stability balls. In addition, every exercise you perform should be multi-joint, using many different muscle groups at the same time. This maximizes the efficiency of your workout time and also results in a much greater anabolic, muscle-building hormone release compared with single-joint exercises that target just one muscle group.

The following full body workout should ideally be performed three days per week, with at least 24 hours of recovery between each workout. Depending on how much time you have available and your starting fitness level, you can do from two to five sets in the workout. Be sure to choose challenging weights, although you can perform a "warm-up" set with lighter weights for each exercise if you have time. Rather than doing all sets for each exercise before moving to the next exercise, this workout is a multi-round circuit that progresses from exercise to exercise. This will allow you to save time and still add muscle.

If you cannot complete a set using the weight you've chosen for that exercise, stop, rest a few seconds, then keep going with that same weight. As long as you can maintain good form, it's always better for you to choose heavier rather than lighter weights.

In addition, you will find two additional workouts below the main workout. These are optional, but are highly recommended, and are meant to be performed on the days between your main workouts or on a weekend day. For example, you could do the workout below on Monday, Wednesday, and Friday, then do the two additional workouts on Tuesday and Thursday.

For a detailed explanation of sets, reps, tempo, load, and other weight training tips, go to "Definitions" in the Appendix (p. 135). You can print workouts to take to the gym with you at GetFitGuy.com.

△ *Male Ectomorph Full Body Workout*

EXERCISE	SETS	REPS	TEMPO	LOAD
Warm-up: Complete 3–5 minutes of aerobic exercise such as jogging, cycling, or using an elliptical trainer. Or complete the warm-up program in the Appendix of this book (p. 141).				
Main Set: Complete the following exercises as a circuit, two to four times through, with a recovery of 60–90 seconds after each exercise and a recovery of 2–3 minutes after each set.				
Dumbbell or barbell chest presses, **p. 228**	2–4	6–8	fluent	85–90%
Dumbbell or barbell dead lifts, **p. 216**	2–4	6–8	fluent	85–90%
Dumbbell or barbell cleans, **p. 219**	2–4	6–8	fluent	85–90%
Dumbbell or barbell squats, **p. 211**	2–4	6–8	fluent	85–90%
Dumbbell or barbell overhead push presses, **p. 206**	2–4	6–8	fluent	85–90%
Pull-ups, **p. 242**	2–4	6–8	fluent	85–90%
*Cool-down: Hold each of the following stretches for 6–20 seconds. If heart rate is high or breathing is difficult, complete 3–5 minutes of light aerobic activity prior to the stretches.				
Lunging hip flexor	1	1	control	body
Spiderman	1	1	control	body
Single-leg quadriceps	1	1	control	body
Calf	1	1	control	body
Achilles/foot	1	1	control	body
Standing, seated, or lying hamstring	1	1	control	body
Lying leg cross body	1	1	control	body
Lying leg open body	1	1	control	body

* For these, and many other exercises, go to GetFitGuy.com.

Extra Male Ectomorph Workout 1. Arms and Core

Warm up with 2–5 minutes of easy aerobic exercise (such as jumping jacks, squats, running, bicycling), then complete 5 maximum intensity, 30-second efforts on the elliptical, bike, treadmill, or rowing machine. Next, complete 2–5 rounds of the first two exercises, back to back with minimal rest, before moving on to the next two exercises.

Romanian dead lift with bicep curl—10 reps (p. 217)
Dumbbell kickbacks—10 reps (p. 210)
Cable torso twists—10 reps (p. 230)
Little bigs (hold a weight in your hands)—10 reps (p. 197)

Extra Male Ectomorph Workout 2. Legs and Core

Warm up with 2–5 minutes of easy aerobic exercise, then complete 5 maximum intensity, 30-second efforts on the elliptical, bike, treadmill, or rowing machine. Complete 2–5 rounds of the first two exercises, back to back with minimal rest, before moving on to the next two exercises.

Walking lunges with twist—10 reps (p. 222)
Cable kick backs—10 reps per side (p. 239)
Superman—10 reps (p. 194)
V ups (hold a weight in your hands)—10 reps (p. 196)

Your Nutrition Tips

As you learned earlier, your metabolism is incredibly high, and you simply will not be able to add muscle to your skinny frame unless you eat a high number of calories from nutrient-dense foods. A nutrient-dense food contains as many vitamins, minerals, and nutrients as possible for each calorie. In other words, it is the complete opposite of an empty calorie food like a doughnut or a piece of white bread. Rather than these quick, starchy calories, you should instead be eating plenty of nuts, dried fruits, seeds, smoothies, coconut milk, avocados, meat, and protein shakes, along with healthy vegetable-based fiber so your digestive tract doesn't get backed up from all those calories. To give you an idea of what a high number of calories would be, I can tell you that I've personally trained male ectomorphs attempting to gain size or to prepare for sports or bodybuilding, and many were eating in excess of 5,000 calories per day!

Although there are some body types that don't need to frequently snack or graze, frequent eating is actually a good strategy for you. If you're a busy person constantly on the go, these snacks can come from fast and easy sources, like smoothies, shakes, bars, or trail mixes. If these type of foods are prepackaged, they should come from unprocessed natural ingredients with few preservatives, such as fruit, nuts, seeds, coconuts, and healthy protein powders. Finally, for soups and salads, you can add extra calories and flavor with toppings such as oils, seeds, nuts, whole grain or flaxseed crackers or cereal, and cubed or crumbled cheese.

If you're doing the workouts in this book and find that

you're having a difficult time gaining muscle, then there are two possible causes:

1. You're not eating enough food. The best remedy for this is to log what you eat, keeping track of total calories consumed. Often it can feel like you're eating a lot when you are really nowhere close to eating the amount that you actually need.

2. Your testosterone levels are low or you have a testosterone-estrogen imbalance. This is often the case in males over thirty, and is a more complicated issue. I have addressed this topic many times at BenGreenfieldFitness.com, so I'd recommend you go there and do a search for *testosterone*. It's also a good idea to get your hormone levels tested by your doctor.

In addition, if you're trying to accelerate muscle gain, you should go to GetFitGuy.QuickandDirtyTips.com and read the two-part series "Do Muscle-Building Supplements Really Work?"

While controlling large fluctuations in blood sugar is important for health reasons, your body type can handle more carbohydrates than the other body types, and you don't need to avoid or eliminate carbohydrates, despite the message of popular muscle magazines that preach a high-protein diet. This is not a good strategy for an ectomorph. Instead of cutting out carbs, you simply need to ensure that they come from healthy sources such as sprouted whole grains, rice, quinoa, amaranth, millet, sweet potatoes, yams, taro, beets, or other natural, minimally processed carbohydrate sources.

Finally, if you look at most nutrition labels, they are based on an average 2,000 calories per day. This is not going to be enough for your metabolism and nutritional needs, especially if you are physically active. You can approximate your daily calorie needs (otherwise known as your basal metabolic rate, or BMR) by using the calorie calculator at GetFitGuy.com.

Sample Daily Meal Plan for Male Ectomorph

Breakfast   CEREAL ▸ ½–1 cup cooked quinoa or oatmeal with 2–3 heaping scoops protein powder, 2–3 tablespoons coconut milk or whole yogurt, 1–2 tablespoon almond butter, ½ teaspoon cinnamon, and 1 sliced banana or handful of raisins or berries.

Morning Snack   1 piece fresh fruit, such as a pear, an apple, or a grapefruit with 1–2 tablespoons of peanut or almond butter, or a handful of nuts, preferably raw almonds, macadamia nuts, cashews, or Brazil nuts.

Lunch   LARGE WRAP OR SANDWICH ▸ For protein portion, use leftovers from dinner, or 6–8 ounces of sliced turkey, chicken, ground beef, ground buffalo, or nonfried fish. For vegetable options, use peppers, cucumber, tomato, sprouts, red onion, or celery. For extra calories, add ½–1 avocado and a handful of feta cheese. For sauce or dressing options, use olive oil/vinaigrette, yogurt, lemon or lime juice, or a fermented soy sauce.

Smoothie   Blend ice, 1–2 tablespoons almond butter or a handful of raw almonds, 1–2 scoops protein powder, 1 banana, and whole coconut milk to desired texture.

Dinner   SALMON, MACKEREL, HALIBUT, SOLE, OR SNAPPER ▸ Prepare 6–8 ounces with olive oil, garlic, lemon juice, mushrooms, red onions, salt, pepper (or as desired). Serve with roasted or sautéed green beans, asparagus, steamed spinach, or kale seasoned with sea salt, pepper, turmeric to taste, lemon juice, and slivered almonds. Include, if available, 1–2 pinches of parsley, thyme, oregano, and/or basil. Serve with a large sweet potato or 1 cup of cooked white or brown rice, seasoned to taste.

Dessert   HOMEMADE REESE'S PEANUT BUTTER CUP ▶ Use one small container of Greek yogurt. Add 1 tablespoon nut butter and 2 tablespoons dark chocolate pieces or cocoa mix. Stir together, close your eyes, and imagine you just took it out of that little orange wrapper. Freeze for added effect.

CHAPTER 9

Body Type: Male Ecto-Mesomorph

In junior high and high school, I was skinny but not slight. I had broad shoulders, but they were bony; I had muscular arms, but not bulging; and I had a flat stomach, but not one that was extremely "ripped." Once college rolled around, I began lifting and playing the explosive sport of tennis and actually developed a fairly impressive physique that I later used for success at bodybuilding. Now, five years later, I'm 30 pounds lighter than I was in those bodybuilding days, and a relatively skinny triathlete. For the most part, I have been able to trigger these significant changes in body shape and muscle size because I am an ecto-mesomorph. At BenGreenfieldFitness.com, you can see and compare pictures of me in my bodybuilding days with pictures of me as relatively "skinny" endurance athlete.

If you're a male ecto-mesomorph, then like me, you have broad shoulders, a narrow waist, thin ankles and wrists, and a

V-shaped torso. You can easily fluctuate between being incredibly lean or very muscular. Like an ectomorph, when you do gain weight, the fat tends to be on the stomach, but unlike an ectomorph, it can also be on your upper thighs and buttocks. Like a mesomorph, you can quickly build muscle and tend to be fairly athletic, but not quite as powerful or explosive (think of yourself as a swimmer versus a linebacker).

Your natural body shape is a combination of muscular fast twitch muscle and lean slow twitch muscle, and you tend to morph toward one type or the other based on the physical activities that you choose. For example, if you decide to take up running or bicycling, you'll find that you get skinny fairly quickly, but if you begin to engage in heavy weight training or power sports, your body will pack on muscle, especially in the chest, shoulders, and thighs. You can do just fine in both endurance and strength training, but may not excel in either—which means that a combination of these types of activities is a perfect workout program for you. Often, male ecto-mesomorphs bounce from sport to sport, as we can quickly adapt to multiple exercise forms (but unfortunately this tendency can make it difficult to become skilled at just one sport).

You have a high metabolism and your appetite is fairly strong, but unlike an ectomorph, you gain weight when you indulge in unhealthy foods and can't eat whatever you want without expecting to see fat deposits appear on your stomach, alongside your waist, and on your upper legs. Male ecto-mesomorphs tend to do well on a relatively well balanced mix of slow-burning carbohydrates (such as beans and lentils), natural proteins, and healthy fats.

The kind of muscle that you build is lean and defined, and

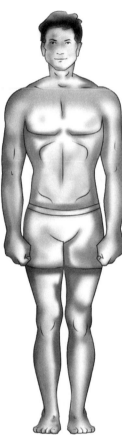

even if you are lifting heavy weights and focusing on muscle gain, you don't usually have bulging muscles that people notice even if you are wearing a sweater or loose shirt. Celebrity examples of male ecto-mesomorphs include actors Hugh Jackman and Christian Bale, and basketball player Dwayne Wade.

Your Strengths

As you can imagine, it comes in handy to be able to easily redefine your body and muscle composition based on the look that you are attempting to achieve, especially if you like a variety of different sports or physical activities or you're interested in acting or modeling. Because of this ability, you can choose to focus on triathlon, tennis, bodybuilding, fashion, and a broad range of other activities that other body types may have more difficulty adapting to.

Because your body fat is relatively low, your chest and shoulders are broad, your waist is naturally narrow and thin, and your legs are long but powerful, you can develop an impressive physique without getting too bulky or heavy, and you will look good in a wide variety of clothing types. If you have a trouble spot or specific area you'd really like to work on, your body responds well to specific exercises targeting that one spot.

Your Limitations

In some ways, it may sound as if you have won the lottery by having a male ecto-mesomorph body. After all, who wouldn't want to be able to easily flip the switch between being thin and being bulked up? But this can also be a disadvantage. You may find it hard to ever get extremely lean (for example, if you wanted to be a competitive runner) or very big (say, if you wanted to have the extra mass necessary for football). So you may never be proficient at a single sport or physical activity, but can be pretty good at all of them.

In addition, while your appetite may be just as raging as a male ectomorph, you can easily put on extra fat, especially in your stomach and upper legs, so while you can certainly get away with eating more than mesomorphs or endomorphs, you do need to be careful about the source of your calories, and choose healthier options skewed toward slow-burning carbohydrates and healthy fat and protein intake.

Finally, because you have a larger frame and bigger bones than an ectomorph, if you lose too much weight (which can easily happen if you exercise a lot and don't eat enough), you can look bony, especially in the shoulders and hips.

Your Ideal Body

If you think your chest and shoulders look embarrassingly bony, then you'll be happy to know that with the right workout and nutrition program, you can add muscle and fill out these areas very quickly. This broad look in your upper body can be combined with an impressively thin waist with defined abdominal musculature.

Although your arms are long and lean with skinny wrists, they have the potential to fill out nicely, especially in the upper arms (biceps and triceps). This, combined with the broad chest and shoulders, can make you look very good in T-shirts without having freakishly venous or overly muscular, bulging arms.

If you are not physically active or don't do lower body exercising, your butt and upper thighs will look lean and skinny, but you can easily fill these areas out with muscle and form an impressive taper from your thighs down to your naturally thin calves and ankles. Although he has a combination of incredible genetic talent and years of training, Olympic sprinter Usain Bolt is one example of a male ecto-mesomorph who is not overly muscular but has an athletic physique—and you can achieve this type of look with the proper combination of endurance and weight training.

Your Workout Plan

Compared to the other body types, you get to have the greatest flexibility and variety in your workout program. To take advantage of your unique combination of slow twitch and fast twitch muscle fibers, you should include elements of strength, power, endurance, and sprinting in your exercise plan.

To get your dream body, you definitely need to be doing some type of weight training or resistance routine at least three times a week. You should choose full body, multi-joint exercises combined with single-joint "vanity" exercises to focus on specific muscle groups that you want to target. The weights that you use should be a combination of light and heavy. It will work well for you to warm up with lighter weights and gradually progress to heavier weights as you move through a workout circuit or sets for a specific exercise. For example, if you were going to do four repeats (sets) of each exercise, your first set or circuit could be 12–15 repetitions, your second 10–12 repetitions, and your third and fourth 8–10 repetitions. Compared with single-joint exercises such as biceps curls, or "body split" style workouts that work specific muscle areas on specific days, a full body weight training program will get you highly desirable results.

In addition to this type of weight training program, you should also perform a combination of aerobic endurance training combined with faster, higher intensity cardiovascular intervals. If you are more interested in a physical activity that requires endurance, you should skew your cardio toward the aerobic workouts, but if you want to excel in sprint sports (or not lose too much weight), you should instead prioritize higher intensity cardio bouts.

For the workouts below, you have your choice of three different weight training programs that you should space 48 hours apart during the week. Depending on your goals, you can then choose an endurance training routine or cardiovascular interval routine to do at a different time of day than your weight training workouts, as a warm-up to your weight training workouts, or on the days between your weight training workouts.

For a detailed explanation of sets, reps, tempo, load, and other weight training tips, go to "Definitions" in the Appendix (p. 135). You can print workouts to take to the gym with you at GetFitGuy.com.

EXERCISE	SETS	REPS	TEMPO	LOAD
Warm-up: Complete 3–5 minutes of aerobic exercise such as jogging, cycling, or using an elliptical trainer. Or complete the warm-up program you will find in the Appendix of this book (p. 141).				
Main Set: Complete the following circuit of exercises. Rest 60–90 seconds, then repeat, for 2–5 rounds. Beginners should choose a lower number of rounds, while more advanced exercisers can do the higher number. For the first set, do 12–15 repetitions, for the next 2–3 sets do 10–12 repetitions, and for the final 2–3 sets, do 8–10 repetitions.				
Overhead push presses, **p. 206**	2–5	varies	fluent	65–70%
Pull-ups or pull-downs, **p. 242**	2–5	varies	fluent	65–70%
Water-ski rows, **p. 231**	2–5	varies	fluent	65–70%
Single-arm cable chest presses, **p. 237**	2–5	varies	fluent	65–70%
Romanian dead lifts, **p. 217**	2–5	varies	fluent	65–70%
Front plank reaches, **p. 191**	2–5	varies	fluent	body
Vanity Abs 1: Crunches, **p. 195**	2–5	15–20	fluent	body
Vanity Abs 2: Side plank lateral raises, **p. 215**	2–5	12–15	fluent	65–70%
Vanity Arms 1: Dumbbell curls, **p. 207**	2–5	varies	fluent	65–70%
Vanity Arms 2: Cable triceps push-downs, **p. 240**	2–5	varies	fluent	65–70%
Vanity Legs 1: Cable leg kickforwards, **p. 239**	2–5	varies	fluent	65–70%
Vanity Legs 2: Cable leg kickbacks, **p. 239**	2–5	varies	fluent	65–70%

Cool-down: Finish with 3–5 minutes of light aerobic activity such as cycling or brisk walking, followed by a full body stretch. Visit Tinyurl.com/benstretch for a full body-stretching protocol.

△ *Male Ecto-Mesomorph Full Body Workout 2*

EXERCISE	SETS	REPS	TEMPO	LOAD
Warm-up: Complete 3–5 minutes of aerobic exercise such as jogging, cycling, or using an elliptical trainer. Or complete the warm-up program you will find in the Appendix of this book (p. 141).				
Main Set: Complete the following circuit of exercises. Rest 60–90 seconds, then repeat, for 2–5 rounds. Beginners should choose a lower number of rounds, while more advanced exercisers can do the higher number. For the first set, do 12–15 repetitions, for the next 2–3 sets do 10–12 repetitions, and for the final 2–3 sets, do 8–10 repetitions.				
Straight-arm cable pull-downs, **p. 232**	2–5	varies	explosive	65–70%
Walking lunges with twist, **p. 222**	2–5	varies	fluent	65–70%
Cable rows, **p. 230**	2–5	varies	fluent	65–70%
Push-ups, **p. 187**	2–5	varies	fluent	body
Barbell or dumbbell squats, **p. 211**	2–5	varies	fluent	65–70%
Side plank rotations, **p. 216**	2–5	varies	fluent	body
Vanity Abs 1: Crunches, **p. 195**	2–5	15–20	fluent	body
Vanity Abs 2: Side plank lateral raises, **p. 215**	2–5	12–15	fluent	65–70%
Vanity Arms 1: Dumbbell curls, **p. 207**	2–5	varies	fluent	65–70%
Vanity Arms 2: Triceps cable pushdowns, **p. 240**	2–5	varies	fluent	65–70%
Vanity Legs 1: Cable leg kickforwards, **p. 239**	2–5	varies	fluent	65–70%

(continued)

Exercise	Sets	Reps	Tempo	Load
Vanity Legs 2: Cable leg kickbacks, **p. 239**	2–5	varies	fluent	65–70%

Cool-down: Finish with 3–5 minutes of light aerobic activity such as cycling or brisk walking, followed by a full body stretch. Visit Tinyurl .com/benstretch for a full body-stretching protocol.

△ *Male Ecto-Mesomorph Full Body Workout 3**

Exercise	Sets	Reps	Tempo	Load
Warm-up: Complete 3–5 minutes of aerobic exercise such as jogging, cycling, or using an elliptical trainer. Or complete the warm-up program you will find in the Appendix of this book (p. 141).				
Side-to-side leg swings	1	8–10	explosive	body
Front-to-back leg swings	1	8–10	explosive	body
Hip flexor kickouts	1	8–10	explosive	body
Arm swings	1	8–10	explosive	body
Arm circles	1	8–10	explosive	body

* For these, and many other exercises, go to GetFitGuy.com.

EXERCISE	SETS	REPS	TEMPO	LOAD
Main Set: Complete the following circuit of exercises. Rest 60–90 seconds, then repeat, for 2–5 rounds. Beginners should choose a lower number of rounds, while more advanced exercisers can do the higher number. For the first set, do 12–15 repetitions, for the next 2–3 sets do 10–12 repetitions, and for the final 2–3 sets, do 8–10 repetitions.				
Goblet squats, **p. 212**	2–5	varies	fluent	65–70%
Ball leg curls, **p. 227**	2–5	varies	fluent	65–70%
Single-arm dumbbell rows, **p. 209**	2–5	varies	fluent	65–70%
Incline push-ups, **p. 189**	2–5	varies	fluent	body
Cable chest flies, **p. 236**	2–5	varies	fluent	65–70%
Cable torso twists, **p. 230**	2–5	varies	fluent	65–70%
Vanity Abs 1: Crunches, **p. 195**	2–5	15–20	fluent	body
Vanity Abs 2: Side plank lateral raises, **p. 215**	2–5	12–15	fluent	65–70%
Vanity Arms 1: Dumbbell curls, **p. 207**	2–5	varies	fluent	65–70%
Vanity Arms 2: Cable triceps push-downs, **p. 240**	2–5	varies	fluent	65–70%
Vanity Legs 1: Cable leg kickforwards, **p. 239**	2–5	varies	fluent	65–70%
Vanity Legs 2: Cable leg kickbacks, **p. 239**	2–5	varies	fluent	65–70%

Cool-down: Finish with 3–5 minutes of light aerobic activity such as cycling or brisk walking, followed by a full body stretch. Visit Tinyurl.com/benstretch for a full body-stretching protocol.

If your focus is on endurance or limiting any gains in muscle size, then substitute any of the following high intensity cardio interval workouts with 30–60 minutes of easy cardio at a conversational pace, such as jogging, using an elliptical trainer, swimming, or cycling. To further limit muscle gains or accelerate fat loss, do any cardio sessions on an empty stomach in the morning before breakfast. The program you find in this chapter is very similar to what I personally do, with the addition of long cardio sessions on the weekend for my Ironman triathlon training.

High Intensity Cardio Interval Workout 1

> *5-minute warm-up*
>
> *3 minutes at a hard effort, followed by 1 minute very high intensity*
>
> *4 minutes at a moderate pace*
>
> *2 minutes at a hard effort, followed by 1 minute very high intensity*
>
> *3 minutes at a moderate pace*
>
> *1 minute at a hard effort, followed by 1 minute very high intensity*
>
> *2 minutes at a moderate pace*
>
> *3-minute cool-down*

High Intensity Cardio Interval Workout 2

> *5 minutes at a moderate pace*
>
> *3×30 seconds hard to 30 seconds moderate*
>
> *2×1 minute hard to 1 minute moderate*
>
> *1×2 minute hard to 2 minutes moderate*

Repeat steps 2–4 one more time
2-minute cool-down

High Intensity Cardio Interval Workout 3

5 minutes at a moderate pace
3×30 seconds hard to 30 seconds moderate
2×1 minute hard to 1 minute moderate
1×2 minute hard to 2 minutes moderate
Repeat steps 2–4
2-minute cool-down

Your Nutrition Tips

Although you have enough natural muscle and a high enough metabolism to eat a large number of calories, you need to be careful of the source of those calories. Male ecto-mesomorphs eating lots of starchy carbohydrates or junk foods deposit more fat on the stomach and upper legs, and for this reason, most of your diet should come from slow-burning carbohydrates (for example, beans, lentils, nuts, and seeds), natural proteins (wild-caught salmon), and healthy fats (avocados and olives). If you want to shed muscle and are going for a lean look, you would also benefit from experimenting with a vegan or vegetarian diet (I personally lost 10 pounds of muscle with just 6 weeks of raw, vegan eating).

You don't need to snack between meals if you are eating three large meals per day. But you may find that you experience appetite cravings and choose the wrong foods for your main meals if you don't include snacks. For this reason, try to have at least two healthy snacks on hand during the day—one for between breakfast and lunch and another for between lunch and dinner. Use the strategy of carbohydrate timing, which means that breakfast and your first snack of the day should be more carbohydrate rich, since your metabolism will be higher early in the day. This will also give you the energy you need for your workouts. Your afternoon snack should be more fat-based, with healthy fats that contain high levels of omega-3 fatty acids (like walnuts), monounsaturated fats (like olives), and medium chain triglycerides (like coconut-based foods).

If you need help determining exactly how many calories you should eat for your height and weight, please refer to GetFitGuy.com/calculator for a calorie calculator.

Sample Daily Meal Plan for Male Ecto-Mesomorph

Breakfast   POWER CEREAL ▶ ½–1 cup cooked quinoa or oatmeal with 2–3 heaping scoops of protein powder, 2–3 tablespoons of coconut milk or whole yogurt, 1–2 tablespoons of almond butter, ½ teaspoon of cinnamon, and 1 sliced banana or a handful of raisins or berries.

Morning Snack   1 piece fresh fruit (e.g., a grapefruit or an apple). For extra calories, add a handful of pumpkin seeds or Brazil nuts.

Lunch   PROTEIN SALAD ▶ Over a bed of mixed greens, kale, or any other dark leafy green, add ½–1 avocado, ½–1 can of sardines in olive oil (or 4–6 ounces of any other meat of choice), a small handful of feta cheese, a handful of olives, a sliced tomato, and any other sliced or chopped vegetables of choice. Use olive oil and balsamic vinaigrette as dressing, or just use the oil from the sardines. If you are exercising in the afternoon, you can include a small portion of carbs with lunch, such as serving your salad over ½ cup of cooked brown rice, or include white or black beans as a salad topping.

Afternoon Snack   Coconut milk mixed with protein powder, banana, and almond butter.

Dinner   BAKED SALMON WITH ROASTED VEGETABLES AND POTATOES ▶ In a shallow baking dish, coat baby red potatoes with olive oil and salt and roast for 10–12 minutes, until they begin to brown on the bottom. Turn the potatoes over and roast another 10 minutes until browned on top. Remove the baking dish from the oven, then add vegetables of choice (asparagus, red onions, or chopped red peppers work well) that have been tossed with garlic, salt, and olive oil. Add the vegetable mixture to the potatoes and stir to combine, then add a large filet of salmon and return the baking dish to the oven for 10 minutes, or until the fish is cooked through.

Extra Snack   Fat and protein-based energy bar, such as a CocoChia Snack Bar, a BumbleBar, or a Hammer Bar.

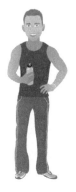

CHAPTER 10

Body Type: Male Mesomorph

Ancient warriors, superheroes, football stars—the male meso-morph is often personified in literature, comics, and sports as the ultimate macho type. Mesomorphs are thought of as gene-tically gifted, with a body that looks good and excels at athlet-ics. Many of the world's top athletes, bodybuilders, weight lifters, and action stars are mesomorphs, including Michael Phelps, Mark Wahlberg, Dwayne "The Rock" Johnson, Sylves-ter Stallone, Bruce Willis, and LL Cool J.

If you are a mesomorph, you are naturally muscular and have a thick, athletic build with medium-sized bones. You likely have a strong, defined jaw, a round, slightly barrel-shaped chest, a rectangular, muscular waist, large arms, and thick thighs and calves. However, even though your upper body is wide, you don't quite have the same V shape as a male ecto-mesomorph, and since your waist is a bit more rectangular

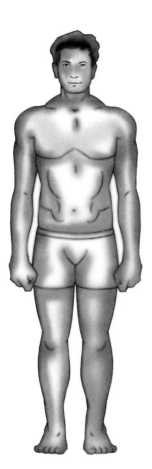

(without the sharp taper in at the waist) you tend to have a more square appearance.

If you're in good shape and your body fat is low, your abdominals are well defined—a classic six-pack or even eight-pack. However, your stomach area is one of the first places you'll tend to put on fat if you gain weight. Your legs are muscular, with thick buttocks and thighs, trouble spots for depositing fat if you gain significant weight. Your lower legs are relatively thinner, but still defined. Your chest and upper back can also get flabby if you aren't careful.

Your metabolism is not as high as that of an ectomorph or ecto-mesomorph, so you have to be careful what you eat, especially as you age or you are less active. Many older male mesomorphs gain weight due to the natural decline in muscle over time. So if you don't want to look like that athletic guy who got fat, then you should up healthy eating and exercise activities as early in life as possible.

Fortunately, you will find that losing fat and gaining muscle is easy for you. You respond very quickly to exercise, in your ability both to gain cardiovascular fitness and muscle and to lose weight or target trouble spots. Thus you can develop your ideal body very efficiently if you have the proper workout and nutrition program.

Your Strengths

Since you gain muscle mass and lose weight quickly, you can achieve fitness and definition efficiently, and you respond well to relatively small doses of exercise. In particular, you can develop impressive chest, shoulder, arm, and abdominal muscles, and if you stay lean, muscular and defined legs as well. The key for you is to lower your body fat percentage several points, which then allows you to take advantage of your considerable lean muscle mass.

With your natural athleticism, sports that involve sprinting, shoving, weight lifting, jumping, or power are all naturally easier for you. So when it comes to popular team sports such as basketball, baseball, or football, you have won the DNA lottery. Depending on your amount of muscle mass, you can be good at endurance-based sports as well, but these activities usually require male mesomorph body types to be at a relatively low weight, which might be tough for you to achieve and maintain.

Your Limitations

The biggest barrier in your physical appearance is keeping your body fat percentage low enough to actually show off your muscle definition. Since you gain fat as easily as you gain muscle, you need to be consistent with exercise, and also careful with your total calorie intake and carbohydrate consumption. Your weight fluctuates, which can lead to frustrating yo-yo cycles of fat gain and loss.

Your lower body has more trouble spots than your upper body, and if you are overweight, you'll find that your buttocks and thighs tend to get thick and bulky. This means that you can go up in pant sizes very quickly if you aren't staying active and watching your diet.

Your body type is best suited to strength and power, so

jogging, cycling, swimming, and other endurance activities can be tough—and you may find it frustrating if you train hard for a bike ride, marathon, or other long sporting event and yet are easily passed by ectomorphs or ecto-mesomorphs who don't seem to be huffing and puffing nearly as hard as you. Part of this is because muscle can be difficult to cool and carry, and also because your square body shape is biomechanically better at producing large amounts of force over a short period of time, rather than small amounts of force over a long period of time.

Your Ideal Body

Of all the ideal bodies I've written about in this book, yours is the easiest to describe because it is so often typified in pop culture as the ultimate shape for a man. Just glance at the cover of nearly every men's fitness and health magazine, and you will be looking at a typical (though likely airbrushed) version of the dream body for a male mesomorph. Drawings of superheroes such as Batman and Superman also typify what the male mesomorph body can look like when in good shape.

Your chest has clean definition and appears to have a sharp 90-degree angle cut from the top to the sides. The triangular deltoid muscle on either shoulder juts sharply out to the side when your upper body is in shape. This, combined with the lack of a significant inward cut of the waist in your naturally muscular abdominals, is what primarily contributes to your powerful, square-shaped appearance.

Your arms are naturally muscular and tend to form bulges and veins when you get into good shape—in other words, it's easy for you to get guns. Your rectus abdominis, the primary muscle that runs down the front of your stomach, has deeper muscle lines that allow for a defined six- or eight-pack, depending on your natural genetics.

Although your butt and thighs do tend to be slightly bulkier, if you include properly structured cardiovascular exercise and regular sporting activities in your routine, you can keep your upper legs low in body fat, muscularly defined, and in proportion to the rest of your body. Your lower legs build muscle quickly, and if you're including movements like running, squats, and lunges in your program, you don't even need to do any specific lower body movements, such as calf raises.

Your Workout Plan

As a male mesomorph, you naturally maintain higher amounts of lean muscle fiber, and compared to the other body types, it isn't necessary for you to do a significant number of multi-joint, full body lifts.

Because of this, your workout plan should be a body part split program, which includes chest, shoulders, and abs on day 1, upper back and arms on day 2, and legs, lower back, and abs on day 3. You'll have three options for your weekly regimen:

1. Do each of these workouts once, for a total of three weight training sessions per week.
2. Do each of these workouts twice, for up to six days of weight training per week.
3. Do each of these workouts once, and then repeat only the workouts that target your trouble spots (such as doing the legs twice a week and the upper body only once).

Unless you're competing heavily in sports, you don't need to focus much on lower repetition, higher weight, or strength or power sets, and can instead perform a medium number of sets (3–4) with a moderate weight and a repetition range of 10-15. Don't burn yourself out by long marathon bouts of exercise at the gym. Rather than doing long workouts a few times a week, split long workouts into two-a-days, or simply exercise for a shorter period of time every day of the week.

If you want to keep your body fat low and improve muscle definition, your program should include one to two long, slow fat-burning cardio sessions. Also, to increase or maintain cardiovascular fitness and lung capacity, you should include one to two high intensity cardio interval sessions. These cardio sessions can be done before, after, or at a different time of day from your weight training.

Below, you will find a male mesomorph body part split program, with two upper body workouts and one lower body workout—each of which use back-to-back supersets to maximize your workout efficiency. To keep your muscles responding to your workouts, switch up exercises every four weeks. You can find variations for each of the body parts at GetFitGuy .com. You'll also have two choices for high intensity interval training workouts and a long, slow fat-burning cardio session.

For a detailed explanation of sets, reps, tempo, load, and other weight training tips, go to "Definitions" in the Appendix (p. 135). You can print workouts to take to the gym with you at GetFitGuy.com.

△ *Male Mesomorph Workout 1: Chest, Shoulders, and Abs*
(Do 1–2 times a week.)

EXERCISE	SETS	REPS	TEMPO	LOAD
Warm-up: Complete 3–5 minutes of aerobic exercise such as jogging, cycling, or using an elliptical trainer. Or complete the warm-up program in the Appendix of this book, (p. 141).				
Superset 1: Complete the following exercises back to back with minimum rest. Rest 60–90 seconds, then repeat, for 2–4 sets. Beginners should choose a lower range of sets, while more advanced exercisers can do the higher range.				
Dumbbell chest presses, **p. 228**	2–4	10–12	fluent	75–80%
Cable flies, **p. 236**	2–4	10–12	fluent	75–80%
Superset 2: Complete the following exercises back to back with minimum rest. Rest 60–90 seconds, then repeat, for 2–4 sets.				
Cable chest presses, **p. 236**	2–4	10–12	fluent	75–80%
Push-ups, **pp. 187–90**	2–4	10–12	fluent	body
Superset 3: Complete the following exercises back to back with minimum rest. Rest 60-90 seconds, then repeat, for 2–4 sets.				
Dumbbell overhead press, **p. 205**	2–4	10–12	fluent	75–80%
Dumbbell side raises, **p. 208**	2–4	10–12	fluent	75–80%
Superset 4: Complete the following exercises back to back with minimum rest. Rest 60–90 seconds, then repeat, for 2–4 sets. You can choose any flexing/extending exercises for lower body.				

EXERCISE	SETS	REPS	TEMPO	LOAD
Cable torso twists, **p. 230**	2–4	10–12	fluent	75–80%
Side plank rotations, **p. 216**	2–4	10–12	fluent	body

Cool-down: Finish with 3–5 minutes of light aerobic activity such as cycling or brisk walking, followed by a full body stretch. Visit Tinyurl.com/ benstretch for a full body-stretching protocol.

△ Male Mesomorph Workout 2: Upper Back and Arms
(Do 1–2 times a week.)

EXERCISE	SETS	REPS	TEMPO	LOAD
Warm-up: Complete 3–5 minutes of aerobic exercise such as jogging, cycling, or using an elliptical trainer. Or complete the warm-up program in the Appendix of this book (p. 141).				
Superset 1: Complete the following exercises back to back with minimum rest. Rest 60–90 seconds, then repeat, for 2–4 sets. Beginners should choose a lower range of sets, while more advanced exercisers can do the higher range.				
Pull-ups or pull-downs, **p. 242**	2–4	10–12	fluent	75–80%
Reverse pull-ups or pull-downs, **p. 242**	2–4	10–12	fluent	75–80%

(continued)

Exercise	Sets	Reps	Tempo	Load
***Superset 2**: Complete the following exercises back to back with minimum rest. Rest 60–90 seconds, then repeat, for 2–4 sets.*				
Seated rows, **p. 234**	2–4	10–12	fluent	75–80%
Single-arm dumbbell rows, **p. 209**	2–4	10–12	fluent	body
***Superset 3**: Complete the following exercises back to back with minimum rest. Rest 60–90 seconds, then repeat, for 2–4 sets.*				
Triceps push-downs, **p. 240**	2–4	10–12	fluent	75–80%
Cable kickbacks, **p. 239**	2–4	10–12	fluent	75–80%
***Superset 4**: Complete the following exercises back to back with minimum rest. Rest 60–90 seconds, then repeat, for 2–4 sets. You can choose any flexing/extending exercises for lower body.*				
Dumbbell biceps curls, **p. 207**	2–4	10–12	fluent	75–80%
Uppercuts, **p. 206**	2–4	10–12	fluent	75–80%
***Cool-down**: Finish with 3–5 minutes of light aerobic activity such as cycling or brisk walking, followed by a full body stretch. Visit Tinyurl.com/benstretch for a full body-stretching protocol.*				

△ *Male Mesomorph Workout 3: Legs, Lower Back, and Abs*
(Do 1–2 times a week.)

EXERCISE	SETS	REPS	TEMPO	LOAD
Warm-up: Complete 3–5 minutes of aerobic exercise such as jogging, cycling, or using an elliptical trainer. Or complete the warm-up program in the Appendix of this book (p. 141).				
Superset 1: Complete the following exercises back to back with minimum rest. Rest 60–90 seconds, then repeat, for 2–4 sets. Beginners should choose a lower range of sets, while more advanced exercisers can do the higher range.				
Dumbbell or barbell squats, **p. 211**	2–4	10–12	fluent	75–80%
Cable leg kickforwards, **p. 239**	2–4	10–12	fluent	75–80%
Superset 2: Complete the following exercises back to back with minimum rest. Rest 60–90 seconds, then repeat, for 2–4 sets.				
Walking lunges, **p. 213**	2–4	10–12	fluent	75–80%
Ball leg curls, **p. 227**	2–4	10–12	fluent	body
Superset 3: Complete the following exercises back-to-back with minimum rest. Rest 60–90 seconds, then repeat, for 2–4 sets.				
Lateral lunges, **p. 198**	2–4	10–12	fluent	75–80%
Cable adduction, **p. 238**	2–4	10–12	fluent	75–80%

(continued)

EXERCISE	SETS	REPS	TEMPO	LOAD
Superset 4: Complete the following exercises back to back with minimum rest. Rest 60–90 seconds, then repeat, for 2–4 sets. You can choose any flexing/extending exercises for lower body.				
Ball back extensions, **p. 226**	2–4	10–12	fluent	75–80%
Ball pikes, **p. 224**	2–4	10–12	fluent	75–80%
Cool-down: Finish with 3–5 minutes of light aerobic activity such as cycling or brisk walking, followed by a full body stretch. Visit Tinyurl.com/ benstretch for a full body-stretching protocol.				

In addition to the weight training workouts above, you should complete the high-intensity cardio intervals below one to two times per week. You can do them before or after your weight training session, at a different time of day from your weight training session, or on a completely separate day. In addition, one to two times per week you should perform 30–60 minutes of easy cardio, such as jogging, using an elliptical trainer, swimming, or cycling. Try to do the easy cardio on an empty stomach in the morning before breakfast, as this can help to accelerate fat loss.

High Intensity Cardio Interval Workout 1

5-minute warm-up

2 minutes at a very hard effort, followed by 1 minute very high intensity

Repeat 2 minutes at a very hard effort, followed by 1 minute very high intensity 6–10 times

3–5 minutes of cool-down

High Intensity Cardio Interval Workout 2

5 minutes at a moderate pace

3×30 seconds hard to 30 second moderate

2×1 minute hard to 1 minute moderate

1×2 minute hard to 2 minutes moderate

Repeat steps 2–4 one more time

3–5 minutes of cool-down

Your Nutrition Tips

Since the mesomorph appetite is not as raging as that of the ectomorph or ecto-mesomorph, you really don't need to snack much and can get away with three square meals a day. These meals should be skewed toward protein. Frequent snacking can add unnecessary calories, keep your blood sugar levels relatively high, and inhibit your body's ability to burn fat. The only exception to this is that before or after your workouts, you should include a small snack to assist with energy and recovery.

Because of your relatively slower metabolism, you should choose natural proteins (fish and healthy fats such as seeds and nuts) instead of carbohydrates or energy-dense foods. In order to feel the most energy and experience the best recovery after you workouts, fuel your naturally higher percentages of lean muscle fiber with consistent, high-quality protein.

Male mesomorphs can quickly and easily gain fat if they don't pay attention to how much they are eating, so write down what you eat or log your diet using online software, a phone app, or a notebook. If you're older, an ex-athlete, or not quite as active as you may have been during other parts of your life, you simply can't get away with eating as many calories as you did when you were more physically active. For male meso-morphs, this can be a difficult adjustment, but caloric control can help you achieve and maintain your dream body for life.

If you need help determining exactly how many calories you should eat, please refer to GetFitGuy.com/calculator for a calorie calculator. This will give you a ballpark figure, although you still need to pay attention to your body and hunger levels, especially if you are doing all the weight training and cardio intervals in this chapter.

Sample Daily Meal Plan for Male Mesomorph

Breakfast   GREEK OMELET ▸ Whisk 3–4 eggs with a splash of milk or cream, then add to a skillet preheated with butter, coconut oil, or olive oil. When bubbles form, add spinach, chopped red onions, gar-lic (optional), and feta cheese. Then use a spatula to fold om-elet. Cook for 2–4 minutes. Serve with sliced tomato, sea salt, and olive oil.

Lunch   WRAP ▸ Into a sprouted whole grain wrap, add 4–6 ounces of low-sodium, low-preservative deli turkey or roast beef, 2–3 slices cheese of choice, ½–1 avocado, spinach or lettuce, chopped olives, sprouts, and any other vegetable of choice. Serve with 1 piece of fresh fruit, such as a pear.

Pre or Post-Workout Snack   ENERGY BAR OR SHAKE ▸ Choose an energy bar of 300–450 calories with 15–30 grams of protein and as few artificial sweeteners or sugars as possible, or simply blend whey protein, almond or peanut butter, ice, and coconut milk.

Dinner   STIR-FRY ▸ Sauté 6–8 ounces of beef, pork, or chicken in olive oil, coconut oil, or butter with frozen stir-fry vegetables or chopped handfuls of your favorite vegetables, such as green beans, carrots, cauliflower, spinach, celery, and mushrooms. Season with a low-sodium soy or teriyaki sauce. For added calories, stir in heated peanut butter or almond butter (especially good if you also add cayenne pepper and lemon juice). Serve over ½–1 cup of a cooked grain such as quinoa, amaranth, millet, or white or brown rice.

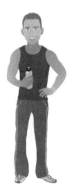

CHAPTER 11

Body Type: Male Endomorph

Imagine my surprise when during an Ironman triathlon, I am easily passed by a shorter, rounder triathlete who is steamrolling along. As if that doesn't make me feel bad enough, this same male endomorph who passes me in the race also looks like he could beat me soundly at weight training, football, or any other power and strength sport. This has happened to me multiple times during triathlons, and highlights a key characteristic of the male endomorph body type—an impressive combination of both cardiovascular endurance and strength.

Because you can burn fat very efficiently, you're good at long, slow cardiovascular exercise such as jogging or cycling. But because you also gain muscle easily, you tend to be naturally strong or powerful as well.

At the same time, you have the most difficulty losing weight and require a combination of close attention to nutrition and

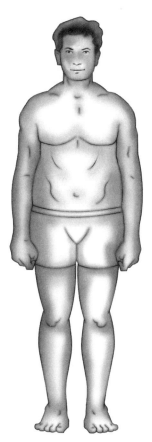

frequent modifications of workout volume and intensity to maintain fat loss. Since your metabolism is naturally slower, you have to be consistent in your workout routine to see results, and you must use ever-changing combinations of cardio, high-intensity interval training, and strength training. Of course, your innate ability to be skilled at multiple modes of exercise can be a great motivation to get to the gym—since you'll obtain the best results from a mix of everything!

As a male endormorph, you have rounder body and are typically shorter (although there are tall endomorphs, such as Alec Baldwin). You are the most curvaceous of the male types, with big bones, a short neck, narrow shoulders, a thick waist, and thick calves and ankles. Your body fat percentage is naturally higher, and you gain fat easily and lose weight slowly.

If your body fat is evenly distributed across your upper and lower body, you have an apple shape, and if you carry more weight in your buttocks, thighs, and upper hips, you have a pear shape. If you're an apple shape, you'll find that you gain and lose muscle and body fat evenly, and if you're a pear shape, you'll notice more muscle and body fat gains and losses in your lower hips and upper legs.

Although celebrity male endomorphs are more popularly cast as the barrel-of-fun characters, when in shape, the endomorph body can cut an impressive figure of power and strength. Just check out Russell Crowe in *Gladiator* or Alec Baldwin in *Miami Blues*. Of course, you can also see examples of less in-shape male endomorphs when you Google Seth Rogen, Cee-Lo Green, Jack Black, and Jon Favreau.

Your Strengths

You are able to develop lean mass with relative ease, which can be a great way to speed up your slightly slower metabolism, burn fat, and achieve your ideal body.

You're an efficient fat burner, and when you get into shape and aren't eating a high carbohydrate diet, you can train your body to go long periods of time on relatively few calories as you burn your storage fat as fuel. Because of this, you actually need to be careful not to eat too few calories, which can leave you sluggish, low on energy, and with an even more depressed metabolism; be careful with crash diets.

Male endomorphs are good at both long, slow bouts of cardio and strength sports such as power lifting or strongman activities. Because of this, you can be excellent at playing football and at running marathons. This is why many endomorphs who've lost significant weight successfully compete in activities such as the Ironman triathlon!

Your Limitations

Because of your sluggish metabolism, you will have a harder time losing weight than the other body types. Your naturally higher body-fat percentage means that you may need to exercise for a longer period of time before you actually see muscle tone and definition. It isn't impossible for you to get your dream body; you simply have to be consistent with both exercise and nutrition planning and execution. You gain fat quickly if you eat the wrong types of foods, or even just slightly more than you actually need, so it can be tough for you to lose weight through diet alone.

That's why exercise is crucial to your achieving your dream body.

Even though you're good at cardiovascular exercise, if you're overweight, activities such as running or cycling feel much harder than they should. But as you shed pounds and lower your body fat percentage, cardio will become more comfortable for your joints and lungs.

Your Ideal Body

With the proper combination of cardio and weights, you can reverse your slow metabolism, pack on fat-burning lean muscle, and significantly lower your body-fat percentage. As you lose weight, you'll begin to notice triangular muscles in your shoulders and a tight, toned look to your chest. Although your arms will always have a slightly higher body fat percentage than those of the other body types, you can develop impressive guns if you're doing the right weight training program.

When a male endomorph loses weight and gets into shape, his abs, stomach, and waist develop a strapping and sturdy appearance. Though you may have trouble developing the deep indentations and the cut look of a six- or eight-pack, you will instead develop a solid, athletic look to your waistline.

Your lower body is extremely powerful and contains high natural amounts of lean muscle mass. A significant drop in body fat percentage can cause the rippling muscles in your thighs, butt, and calves to be quite impressive. If there's any body type to which the term "strong like bull" applies, it is a male endomorph who gets into good shape, since you will look and be physically powerful.

Because of your naturally higher percentage of body fat, you will never achieve the low body-fat percentage and narrow shape of an ectomorph. The key is instead for you to achieve your dream body by burning your fat stores while toning and strengthening your upper half. When this is achieved, you become tight, toned, and compact while still maintaining a very strong look.

Your Workout Plan

Since you burn fewer calories on a regular basis, your entire workout program should be structured around consistent fat-burning cardiovascular exercise, with additional weight training circuits for extra fat loss, and heavier weight training sets for developing your natural strength and a higher level of fat-loss hormones. Single-joint exercises such as biceps curls and triceps extensions, or spot-reducing exercises such as crunches, are extremely *ineffective* for the endomorph body type, and should not be a part of your routine.

Because of your lower metabolic rate, you must exercise consistently, and because you're doing so many different types of exercise, you should try to distribute your sessions evenly throughout as many days of the week as possible. Your longer cardio fat-burning sessions should be performed on an empty stomach, in a fasted state, such as immediately in the morning prior to breakfast. For your other higher intensity workouts that burn more carbohydrate, you'll need to inject strategic snacks, so your metabolism stays elevated.

If you are overweight, choose a mode of cardiovascular exercise that is easy on your hips, knees, and ankles. Instead of pounding away on the treadmill, pick the elliptical trainer, cycling, hiking, power walking, water aerobics, or swimming. Because your male-endomorph body adapts very quickly to the demands you place on it, switch up these cardio modes as often as possible. For example, if on Mondays you do your cardio sessions as a brisk walk or a jog, you may want to switch to bicycling or elliptical on Wednesday or Friday.

For weight training, you should be doing a short, full body exercise circuit one to two times per week, with minimal rest between sets, 12–15 repetitions per set, and 2–4 sets per exercise. You should also include a heavier weight training routine consisting of multi-joint, full body movements one to two times per week. You can do these weight training workouts on the same day as your cardio sessions (preferably at a different time of day), or on the days in between your cardio sessions.

You should change up your weight training exercises at least once every four weeks. Remember that as your cardio burns fat, your weight training will be causing slight increases in muscle. Since muscle weighs more than fat, you may find yourself better motivated by tracking decreases in body fat percentage rather than decreases in weight, since your weight may not appear to be significantly declining even though you're losing substantial amounts of fat.

Below, you will find one high rep, low resistance full body weight training circuit with short cardio bursts, and one low rep, high resistance weight training workout. In addition, you'll find intensity recommendations and instructions for your longer, slower cardio sessions.

For a detailed explanation of sets, reps, tempo, load, and other weight training tips, go to "Definitions" in the Appendix (p. 135). You can print workouts to take to the gym with you at GetFitGuy.com.

△ *Full Body Male Endomorph Circuit*
(Do 1–2 times a week.)

EXERCISE	SETS	REPS	TEMPO	LOAD
Warm-up: Complete 3–5 minutes of aerobic exercise such as jogging, cycling, or using an elliptical trainer. Or complete the warm-up program in the Appendix of this book (p. 141).				
Main Set: Complete the following circuit of exercises. Rest 60–90 seconds, then repeat, for 2–4 rounds. Beginners should choose a lower number of rounds, while more advanced exercisers can do the higher number. IMPORTANT: Finish each circuit with a burst of 30–60 seconds of intense cardio (e.g., elliptical or cycling).				
Goblet squats, **p. 212**	2–4	12–15	fluent	70–75%
Dumbbell walking lunges, **p. 213**	2–4	12–15	fluent	70–75%
Cable torso twists, **p. 230**	2–4	12–15	fluent	70–75%
Dumbbell chest presses, **p. 228**	2–4	12–15	fluent	70–75%
Pull-ups or pull-downs, **p. 242**	2–4	12–15	fluent	70–75%
Dumbbell overhead presses, **p. 205**	2–4	12–15	fluent	70–75%
Single-arm dumbbell rows, **p. 209**	2–4	12–15	fluent	70–75%

Cool-down: Finish with 3–5 minutes of light aerobic activity such as cycling or brisk walking, followed by a full body stretch. Visit Tinyurl.com/benstretch for a full body-stretching protocol.

△ *Full Body Male Endomorph Weight Training Set*
(Do 1–2 times a week.)

EXERCISE	SETS	REPS	TEMPO	LOAD
Warm-up: Complete 3–5 minutes of aerobic exercise such as jogging, cycling or elliptical trainer. Or complete the warm-up program in the Appendix of this book (p. 141).				
Main Set: Complete all sets of each of the following exercises before moving on to the next exercise. After you have completed one set of an exercise, do a light walk, jog, jump rope, crunches, or other active recovery activity for 60–90 seconds, and then do your next set. Beginners should choose a lower number of set, while more advanced exercisers can do the higher number.				
Barbell squats, **p. 220**	2–4	6–8	fluent	85–90%
Barbell overhead presses, **p. 220**	2–4	6–8	fluent	85–90%
Barbell dead lifts, **p. 216**	2–4	6–8	fluent	85–90%
Overhead push presses, **p. 206**	2–4	6–8	fluent	85–90%
Barbell cleans and press **p. 219**	2–4	6–8	fluent	85–90%
Cool-down: Finish with 3–5 minutes of light aerobic activity such as cycling or brisk walking, followed by a full body stretch. Visit Tinyurl.com/benstretch for a full body-stretching protocol.				

In addition to the workouts above, you should perform 30–60 minutes of fat-burning cardio on as many days of the week as possible, preferably in the morning, prior to breakfast. Because these sessions are at a slower rate and can be as simple as a brisk walk out your front door, you don't need to worry that you will overtrain your body by doing them every day. Ideally, you should purchase a heart rate monitor so that you can perform these sessions in your maximum fat-burning heart rate zone.

Once you have a heart rate monitor, here's how to accurately find your personalized fat-burning zone:

- Warm up on a bike for 10 minutes.
- Pedal at your maximum sustainable pace for 20 minutes. You should be breathing hard and your legs should be burning, but you should be able to maintain the same intensity for the full 20 minutes.
- Record your average heart rate during those 20 minutes.
- Subtract 20 beats from that heart rate. Add and subtract 3 beats from the resulting number to get a range. That is your peak fat-burning zone.

Here's an example. Let's say your average heart rate was 160 during the 20-minute pedaling session: $160 - 20 = 140$. Then $140 + 3 = 143$, $140 - 3 = 137$. So your peak fat-burning zone is when you have a heart rate of 137 to 143 beats per minute.

Compared with the results that I have obtained from hundreds of individuals in a professional exercise physiology lab with all sorts of gas masks and gadgets, this method obtains accurate fat-burning zone results. But if you did want to have a laboratory test to find your personal fat-burning zone, then you would look for something called an exercise metabolic rate test, also known as a VO_2 max test.

Your Nutrition Tips

The most important concept for you to understand is that since your body fat percentage is naturally higher, your body can easily rely on its own body fat as a steady supply of energy. But there are several things that can keep this from happening, including:

- A very low calorie diet, which can suppress metabolic rate and fat burning.
- Constantly snacking, especially on carbohydrate-rich foods, which can keep your body clinging to its fat reserves.
- Eating too many pre- and post-workout meals, which your body really needs only for the weight training workouts in this book.

You tend to be highly sensitive to carbohydrate intake, so your eating plan should primarily be comprised of a high amount of lower calorie, nutrient-dense vegetables and lean protein, moderate amounts of healthy fats, and lower amounts of strategically timed carbohydrates. Seemingly healthy foods that may not cause weight gain for other body types, such as sweet potatoes or yams, can still be a problem for the male endomorph, which is why a male ectomorph diet will definitely not work for you.

If you need help determining exactly how many calories

you should eat, please refer to GetFitGuy.com/calculator for a calorie calculator. This will give you a ballpark figure, although you still need to pay attention to your body and hunger levels, especially if you are doing all the weight training and cardio intervals in this chapter.

Because of your slower metabolism, you may feel more tired and fatigued, especially if you are overdoing exercise, so try not to go significantly over and above the recommendations you find in this book. You may want to consider using nutritional supplements such as digestive enzymes and probiotics to allow you to get more nutrients, vitamins, and minerals from the foods that you are eating.

If you're watching your calorie intake and following the nutrition plan, but find that you still seem to be putting on body fat, you may want to consider whether you have any hormonal deficiencies or imbalances. An endocrinologist, registered dietitian, or nutritional therapist can help you test, identify, and treat any issues (such as testosterone deficiency) that may be hindering your progress.

Sample Daily Meal Plan for Male Endomorph

Breakfast   PROTEIN SHAKE ▶ Blend 20–30 grams of whey protein powder, or a vegan mix of pea and rice protein powder, with 1 banana, 1 tablespoon peanut or almond butter, and ice, rice milk, almond milk, or light coconut milk to desired texture.

Lunch   VEGGIE WRAP ▶ Use large leaves of cabbage, bok choy, swiss chard, lettuce, or kale, and make 2–4 small wraps. For inside of each wrap, add a small handful of sliced almonds or crumbled cheese, 2–3 slices of a low-sodium, low-preservative deli meat of choice, sliced olives, 1/2–1 avocado, and any other vegetables of choice, such as sliced tomatoes or cucumbers.

Pre- or Post-Workout Snack Yogurt Parfait ▸ One small container of plain yogurt (does not need to be low-fat or fat-free), with a handful of blueberries or raspberries and a handful of almonds, walnuts, or macadamia nuts or a tablespoon of nut butter.

Dinner Steak with Roasted Vegetables ▸ Into a baking pan coated with 1–2 tablespoons olive oil or with nonstick cooking spray, add sliced zucchini, eggplant, bell peppers, onions, and mushrooms. In a jar, combine 1 teaspoon salt and ¼ teaspoon pepper pepper, 3 tablespoons balsamic vinegar, 2 tablespoons olive oil, 2 cloves crushed garlic, and 1 teaspoon rosemary. Shake the jar, then dump over vegetables. Roast at 425°F. for 15 minutes. While vegetables are roasting, coat a steak (6–8 ounces) with sea salt and olive oil, and cook in a skillet or on the grill for about 5–6 minutes per side.

APPENDIX

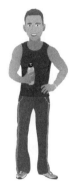

Definitions

If you're a veteran of the gym, you may be able to skip the next several pages. But if you're new to this world, then sets, reps, intensity percentages, and even breathing may all be new concepts to you. Don't worry, all will be made clear in this section.

Breathe

No discussion of exercise basics would be complete without a quick note about proper breathing. During most exercises, blood pressure and overall body tension will increase. If the breath is held during exertion, known as a Valsalva maneuver, the glottis closes and air is blocked from leaving the body, which can significantly increase intra-abdominal pressure and your risk of a hernia, in which the gut contents can be forced through the abdominal wall. Not pretty.

To avoid this risk, breathe out during the most difficult, or exertional, phase of each exercise. Then inhale during the easiest phase of the exercise. For heavier weight lifting and other high intensity activities, such as tennis or baseball, forcefully and rapidly exhale during exertion.

Direction   When a muscle contracts, it shortens in length. This is referred to as a positive or concentric contraction. When a muscle returns to its normal length, it is lengthening. This is referred to as a negative or eccentric contraction. For example, as you bend your elbow, your biceps are shortening, the positive or concentric phase of a biceps curl. As you straighten your elbow, your biceps are returning to their normal length, the negative or eccentric phase of a bicep curl.

Intensity Percentage   There are generally three methods for determining the intensity (or load) of a weight training set. The first method is called 1RM and involves determining the maximum amount of weight that can be lifted for one repetition (this is referred to as your one rep max, or 1RM). Once you have your 1RM, you then determine the number of repetitions that should be performed in a set from certain percentages of that 1RM. This is why you might see someone huffing and puffing to do a single bench press exercise at the gym. They can use the results of that 1RM bench press both to track strength and to extrapolate the weight they should use for higher repetition sets. The table below shows typical repetitions derived from a 1RM.

% LOAD	REPETITIONS
60	17
65	14
70	12
75	10
80	8
85	6
90	5
95	3
100	1

While fairly precise and accurate, the 1RM method is often impractical or even dangerous, since it requires an individual to exert the maximum effort for many different lifts. In addition, you don't really have to track increases in one repetition maximum lift improvements unless you're lifting for competition or engaged in very serious sporting endeavors, such as playing collegiate football. However, if you really want to lift heavy weights, this is a good way to keep track of progress.

The second method for determining intensity is via an equation to derive an approximation of the 1RM. Using this method, you perform a certain number of repetitions for an exercise, then feed that weight and the number of repetitions into an equation to extrapolate what the 1RM load should be. Once the 1RM is approximated, the table above can be used to determine load based on the number of repetitions.

For example, one option is the Brzycki equation:

$$\text{Weight} \div [1.0278 - (0.0278 \times \text{number of repetitions})]$$

An alternative equation is:

$$\text{Weight} \times [1 + (0.033 \times \text{number of repetitions})]$$

At GetFitGuy.com you can find a link to a free max load calculator. The equation method is relatively accurate, provided the number of repetitions used for the equation are 12 or fewer.

The third and final method for determining intensity is by simply using a rating of perceived exertion. When using this method, if an individual can easily lift a weight, the intensity is described as light. If a greater amount of effort is necessary to lift a weight, the intensity is described as medium. If the weight is quite difficult to lift, the intensity is heavy. And if it takes extreme effort to lift the weight, the intensity is described as maximum. The table below can assist with the rating of perceived exertion by comparing to the actual percentage of 1RM.

Intensity as a Percentage of 1RM	Intensity as Rating of Perceived Exertion
70% or less	Light
80%	Medium
90%	Heavy
90% or above	Maximum

Whichever method of determining intensity you use, if you've figured out the load and number of repetitions that you'll be using for a set and you can easily perform the number of repetitions, then you should generally add 5–10 pounds for upper body exercises and 10–20 pounds for lower body exercises.

Rep   A rep, or repetition, is the number of times you actually perform the exercise in one set. For example, one set might include 10, 12, or 15 reps. Typically, the fewer the reps, the higher the intensity or load being moved.

Set   A set is what you do when you perform one specific exercise a certain number of times without stopping to rest. In most workouts of this book, you will repeat a set of an exercise anywhere from two to five times, although some bodybuilders will do up to twenty sets for just one muscle group, which is not recommended unless you like being incredibly sore the next day.

Tempo   The speed or rate of work performed during an exercise will often determine muscle fiber-type recruitment. For example, when a load that is 40 percent of your 1RM is lifted in a slow and controlled manner, primarily slow twitch muscle fibers will be recruited, building muscular endurance. But when that same 40 percent load is lifted in a fast and explosive manner, more motor units and a greater number of fast twitch muscle fibers are recruited, resulting in increased power, strength, or lean muscle development. The tempos used for the workouts in this book are:

Control: Lifting in a slow and controlled manner, with 2–3 seconds for both the directions of the exercise. For example, when you're doing a squat at a control tempo, you should count to three while performing the eccentric (sitting down) phase of the squat, and count to three while performing the concentric (standing up) phase. The control tempo is primarily used for stabilization, injury prevention, or muscle building exercises.

Fluent: Fast yet controlled speed. Typically, the concentric phase of a fluent tempo exercise is 1.5 to 2 times faster than the eccentric phase, since it can be difficult or dangerous for a muscle to move quickly as it lengthens. As an example, in a fluent dumbbell press, the concentric (pressing) phase should be a one count, while the eccentric (lowering) phase should be a two count.

Explosive: As fast as possible in the concentric (or muscle-shortening) phase. Usually, the eccentric (lengthening) phase for an explosive tempo is smooth and controlled, and, 1.5 to 2 times slower than the concentric phase.

Congratulations! You now know more about fancy definitions in weight training than 99 percent of the population. For more advanced tips, such as ways you can alter a set to get more muscle growth, methods to burn more calories with weight training, and other quick and dirty ways to get more out of workouts, check out the Strength Training tab at GetFitGuy .QuickandDirtyTips.com.

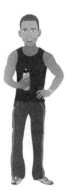

How to Warm Up and Cool Down

Say you're beginning a road trip. You hop in your car, pull it out of the garage, and immediately floor the gas pedal, turn the air-conditioning up high, and blast the radio to full volume. You maintain this same intensity all the way to your final destination, where you abruptly stop, exit your car, slam the door, and walk away. How long do you think your car will handle this sort of abuse before it breaks down? Perhaps you should have slowly progressed into top speed, then given your car a bit of easy driving after intense highway speeds?

Your body is no different from that car. Before you subject it to physical exertion, whether lifting weights, running, bicycling, or playing tennis or golf, you must prepare it for performance. And when you finish your exercise, you must give your body a gradual progression from movement back to sitting in your car, at your desk, or on your couch. In this section, you'll learn why you should warm up and cool down before a workout, and the exercises and stretches—at the right intensity—necessary for a proper warm-up and cooldown.

Why Do I Need to Warm Up Before Exercise?

As you warm up, several positive adaptations take place within your body to prepare you for exercise, including:

- **Dilation of blood vessels**. As your blood vessels dilate or get bigger, your heart doesn't have to work so hard to deliver blood, and you lower your risk of high blood pressure during exercise.
- **Increased temperature**. When you stretch a cold rubber band, it can snap and break. The same is true of muscle. By warming up your muscle tissue, you increase the elasticity and range of motion of your muscles, thus reducing the risk of strains or palls, and you also allow muscles to contract more efficiently. In addition, oxygen in warm blood is more readily available to muscle tissue.
- **Better cooling**. In the same way that the air-conditioning in your car works more efficiently when your car is warmed up, your body's built-in cooling mechanism is optimized when you break a sweat during your warm-up.
- **Hormone production**. As you warm up, your body begins producing hormones like epinephrine, endorphins, growth hormone, and testosterone, all of which increase the energy available for your workout.

- **Mental focus**. Clearing your head with a warm-up allows you to focus more on the difficult or technical movements that will occur during your physical activity, and it also gives you a chance to mentally review your workout, game, or match.

Why Do I Need to Cool Down After Exercise?

As you cool down after the workout, your heart rate slowly returns to normal. That is important, since you're more susceptible to cardiovascular problems when you plop onto the couch or into your car after a workout. When you cool down, you give blood a chance to recirculate throughout your body, which also reduces your risk of fainting and dizziness. A good cool-down also significantly reduces your post-exercise soreness and stiffness.

How to Warm Up Before a Workout

Here are three quick and dirty tips for warming up before a workout:

- **Gradually increase intensity**. If you're going for a run, you can begin with a walk, then move up to a fast walk, then to a jog, and finally to a run. If you're going to lift weights, do a warm-up set with a light weight prior to doing your other sets. If you have time, perform the sample warm-up routine I provide at the end of this chapter.
- **Include range-of-motion exercises**. Interestingly, simply holding a stretch (static stretching) can actually make you

weaker. Additionally, research suggests that static stretching won't really reduce injury risk. Instead, after you've warmed the muscles with cardio movements, do dynamic stretching, which should include arm and leg swings, torso twists, jumping jacks, or fast running. Also include dynamic movement preparation, in which you perform cable or elastic band exercises that move your body through its full range of motion.

- **Activate your brain**. Especially if you're playing sports or doing more advanced exercises, your warm-up should include some balance activities, such as standing on one leg while driving the knee of the opposite leg up to your chest, or closing your eyes and standing on one leg while you do arm swings.

Unless you're a professional athlete, five to ten minutes is enough time for a good warm-up, although the more inactive you are before the workout, the longer the warm-up will need to be.

How to Cool Down After a Workout

Here are your three quick and dirty tips for cooling down after a workout:

- **Gradually decrease intensity**. If you're running, slow down to a jog, then to a brisk walk, and then to a slow walk. If you're lifting weights, save a few of your easier/lighter exercises in the weight room for last.

- **Static stretching**. Holding stretches or doing a few yoga poses after a workout relaxes your body, and the light movements can help with blood flow.
- **Maximize your time**. Doing other activities during your cool-down is fine. For example, you can park your car far away in the gym parking lot and walk to it for your cool-down. You can also catch up on your phone calls with a headset as you stretch or walk, or save any gym social time for your cool-down activities.

A good cool-down should take about five to ten minutes.

Sample Warm-Up and Cool-Down Routine

Warm-up   Arrive at the gym and do a brisk walk for 2 minutes, then progress to a light jog, and finally do a series of three 30-second sprints followed by 30 jumping jacks. Next, lean against a wall and swing each leg 10 times forward and back, then 10 times side to side. Step away from the wall and perform 10 arm circles, then 10 arm swings back and forth.

    Finish with 10 lateral steps to reverse flies in each direction and 10 single-leg row and throws in each direction.

Cool-down   Finish your workout by briskly walking for 2 minutes, then performing a lunging hip flexor stretch with arms overhead, a seated hamstring stretch, and a series of shoulder stretches. Finally, if you have time, use a foam roller for a few minutes. At YouTube.com/BenGreenfieldFitness, you can search for *roller* or *stretch* and see my favorite moves.

The Bottom Line

If you want your body to perform like a used car, then rev it up and floor the gas pedal without preparing it. But if you want your body to last a long time, and be responsive, well-tuned, and always in good working order, use these warm-up and cool-down tips!

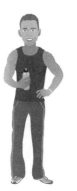

How to Recover After a Workout

Nobody likes to be sore, and at Facebook.com/GetFitGuy I've received many questions about how to eliminate the nagging aches and pains that come from a workout. Though soreness is completely natural and cannot be completely eliminated, it can be controlled, and proper recovery protocols will not only ensure less post-workout discomfort but also allow your body to recover more quickly and benefit more from the workout.

Why Workout Recovery Is Important

Muscles grow and become stronger when they are subjected to forces that cause tiny tears in the muscle fibers. During the recovery period after a workout, the body repairs these fibers and builds new blood vessels to the stressed areas. Additionally, the energy-generating components of the cells develop a higher capacity to work, and bone density increases.

But none of these positive adaptations will occur unless the body rests and recovers. In other words, exercising without recovering properly is a bit like trying to cook a casserole without turning on the oven—you'll go through all the procedures to prepare the casserole but get no final results, or at least a very disappointing final product.

How Sore Should You Be After a Workout?

Excessive soreness is generally an indication that you increased the amount of exercise or the intensity far too quickly in your exercise routine, or that you did not recover properly. Exercise geeks use the term DOMS, which stands for delayed onset muscle soreness; it basically means soreness does not peak immediately after a workout, but instead about 24 to 48 hours post-workout. DOMS that manifests in light muscle tenderness and stiff joints is completely normal, but muscles painful to the touch or sharp pains in the joints are not normal. In other words, if it hurts to twitch, sneeze, giggle, or blink a couple of days after a workout, then you need to pay attention to what you are about to read.

How to Recover After a Workout

Nutrition Immediately after a workout, eat something within the hour. If you do not, you will not have enough carbohydrate energy for your next workout, you will not have enough protein to repair muscles, and you will not have enough fat for hormones and joints. Try a bowl of quinoa or brown rice with chicken, a protein smoothie with whey protein powder and a piece of fruit, or even a slice of last night's pizza.

Hydration   When it comes to recovery, dehydration is one of your biggest enemies, so try to drink one bottle of water for each hour of exercise. A couple hours after a workout, your urine should be light yellow or clear. If it is dark yellow, then you are inadequately hydrated. If it is any other color of the rainbow for that matter, you either need to get glasses or see your physician.

Compression   Performing a brief cool-down after a workout helps muscles milk out excess soreness-generating fluids. Techniques such as massage and a foam roller also help to move inflammatory fluids out of the muscle and also remove adhesions and sore or tight spots. If possible, use a foam roller (My favorite is called "Rumble Roller") once a week or even after every strenuous workout, and schedule a massage once a month. Compression socks and tights can also help and can even be worn during exercise.

Blood flow   Circulation of blood in and out of a stressed body part improves speed of recovery. Techniques that improve blood flow include cooling down after your workout with a walk or easy bike ride, performing light stretching during or after each workout, alternating between hot and cold running water in your post-workout shower, taking an ice bath after a strenuous weight training workout or long run, and performing a light walk, swim, or easy exercise routine the day after a hard workout.

Topical ointments   There are several compounds that you can rub on a muscle to minimize soreness and improve recovery. Most of these compounds work by creating a pain-relieving and cooling sensation, increasing blood flow, or displacing elevated levels of calcium. Popular remedies that have worked for me and my clients include Arnica Rub, Traumeel, BENGAY, Tiger Balm, Dragon Ice, Rock Sauce, and magnesium oil. All of these ointments can be rubbed into the muscle immediately after and up to several days after a workout until soreness subsides.

If you find yourself constantly sore or at a fitness plateau, then use the techniques in this section to recovery properly and get fit more quickly!

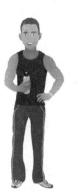

How to Tell If You're Working Out Hard Enough

This section will explain you how to know when your body has had enough exercise to get results, or when it needs more.

How Sore Should You Be After a Workout?

Muscles tear when you exercise, and when they have time to recover properly, they bounce back stronger. While the word *tearing* may sound like a bad thing, it is in fact quite normal, and the tiny micro-tears that occur in a muscle fiber are completely necessary if you actually want to add lean muscle. However, the tearing does cause a little soreness. If you are not a little sore, then you probably did not stimulate your muscles enough to get results.

Yes, that's right, I said a *little* sore, not so sore that you can't move after a workout. If you can't lift a fork to your mouth, turn the steering wheel on your car, or do the dishes, then you have gone too far with your muscle tearing. As a matter of fact, the medical term for excessive muscle tearing is rhabdomyolysis, and this condition results in the release of muscle fiber contents (myoglobin) into the bloodstream. This myoglobin is harmful to the kidneys and can result in kidney damage, extreme fatigue, intense joint and muscle pain, or seizures.

In contrast, you should feel a little sore, but this soreness shouldn't be at the front of your mind. You won't feel like punching a friend in the face if he touches a muscle you exercised the day before, and getting out of bed is not an extreme chore.

So here's my quick and dirty tip for effectively working your muscles. Follow the rule of three. If you can get to the goal number of repetitions for the exercise you are performing, and you can do three or more repetitions over and above your goal number while still maintaining good form, then you should increase the weight you are using. If you cannot get within three repetitions without your eyeballs popping out of your head, you should decrease weight. This rule works very well for workouts in which you're lifting a weight 10–15 times, which is the typical repetition range for most fitness routines.

Contrary to popular belief, while you're weight training, if you feel your muscles burning, this doesn't necessarily indicate that they're being stimulated hard enough to cause tearing or soreness. A burn in your muscles is a result of lactic acid formation and could indicate that you aren't breathing properly. As a matter of fact, try holding your breath while performing a weight lifting set and you'll notice your muscles burn much sooner. This doesn't mean you're working out hard enough to get muscle-stimulating results. It just means your body isn't getting a chance to get rid of carbon dioxide, which is one of the primary ways to buffer lactic acid.

How Should You Feel During Cardio?

While lifting a weight heavy enough to cause muscle tearing and following the rule of three works well for most weight lifting workouts, aerobic exercise requires a different set of criteria. So here are three quick and dirty cardio tips to judge whether you're working out hard enough:

1. Use a heart rate monitor, the monitor on a cardio machine, or your own pulse to track your heart rate during cardio. Find the heart rate at which your muscles begin to burn and you begin to breathe hard. This is your ventilatory threshold heart rate; at this point your body is producing lactic acid and is going into what is called an oxygen debt. Thus you are boosting your metabolism and stimulating cardiovascular fitness and significant calorie burning. Once you have identified this heart rate, attempt to spend 50 percent of your cardio exercise in that zone. One way to do this is to warm up for 5 minutes, then do eight 60-second repeats at ventilatory threshold, with 30 seconds of recovery between each, then move into a 5-minute cool-down.

2. Sweat is a good indicator that your body is attempting to cool itself, meaning that your core temperature and your metabolism have increased. If you're not breaking a sweat, it could mean that you're dehydrated or in a very cold room,

but it is more likely that you need to increase your intensity.

3. Conversational pace means that you can easily carry on a conversation with a friend or workout buddy. During a long, slow cardio routine, a conversational pace is fine. But remember—to become more fit, you can't do all your cardio in that fat-burning zone, so if you're able to carry on a conversation during all your cardio workouts, you're probably not working out hard enough.

How Fast Can You Get Results from a Workout?

Of course the best way to know if you're working out hard enough is whether you're getting the results you desire!

In most cases, after beginning a workout routine or changing a workout routine, you'll notice changes in strength, speed, and performance within just two to four weeks. This is primarily due to your body's ability to learn the new motor patterns and become more efficient at the new movements (and incidentally, is a very good reason to add changes to your workout program every two to four weeks).

But when you're just beginning a workout routine, it can take four to eight weeks to actually notice anatomical changes, such as a flatter stomach, a smaller butt, or a weight loss. So if you've been working out for two months, and you've noticed that you're lifting more weight or going faster on the treadmill, but your body hasn't changed, your enhanced exercise performance is likely the result of improved neuromuscular efficiency, not the result of greater fitness, bigger lungs, or better muscles. If you increase the amount of weight that you lift or the intensity of your workouts, you can actually get results that you see, not just feel.

Finally, remember that if you have a medical condition or you are pregnant, there may be an entirely different set of rules to follow, and you should check with your physician about that before starting a fitness regimen.

The Top 10 Reasons You're Not Losing Weight

Each day I receive several questions from Get-Fit Guy fans. Nearly half are a variation of the same basic question: "Why am I not losing weight?"

Here are the top 10 reasons your body becomes resistant to weight loss and what you can do about it.

10 Reasons You're Not Losing Weight

1. **Stuck in a rut**. There is a principle called SAID, which stands for specific adaptations to imposed demands. Our bodies eventually adapt to the demands we place upon them. If you're doing the same routine week after week or month after month, your body has become very efficient at that routine, and is no longer burning many calories or getting a fitness response. I personally change up my routine every

week, and recommend you introduce new exercises and workouts at least once a month.

2. **Too many calories**. You don't need to frequently snack or consistently fuel your body in order to keep your metabolism elevated. So while it is true that long-term significant calorie deprivation will cause health problems, this shouldn't be used as an excuse to stuff your face and elevate your blood sugar levels every two hours just to boost your metabolism. This strategy usually causes more weight gain and excessive calorie consumption as compared to eating several square meals a day, plus a pre- or post-workout snack.

3. **Not enough calories**. The body needs a specific number of carbohydrates, proteins, and fats in order to sustain metabolism, produce hormones, maintain the immune system, and permit you to have productive workouts. If you're engaging in severe calorie restriction, not only are you sending your body a message to shut down, you're also limiting your ability to productively exercise and potentially damaging your health.

4. **Not lifting weights**. While it may seem counterintuitive, lifting weights actually helps you lose weight. Not only is strength training the best way to replace fat with lean muscle and boost your metabolism, but it also results in a hormonal release that enhances fat loss. Plus, it increases your ability to eat fewer calories without doing damage to the body, since your body can use protein stored in muscle rather than in other vital organs.

5. **Avoiding HIIT**. High intensity interval training, or HIIT, involves intense bouts of cardiovascular exercise, followed by

easy rest periods. Compared to long, slow cardio sessions, HIIT burns far more calories and significantly elevates fat burning. However, the initial discomfort from breathing hard and feeling a full body burn can be daunting. But think about it this way: HIIT allows you to hop on a treadmill and be done in 15–20 minutes. To get the same results with less intense training can require you to slave away on that treadmill for an hour or more!

6. **Low-fat diet**. In the quest to lose fat, it seems logical that you should eat less fat. But if you eat the right kinds of fat, particularly from healthy sources such as avocados, olives, extra virgin olive oil, coconut milk, coconut oil, cold-water fish, seeds, nuts, or yogurt, your body can very efficiently use that fat as a fuel. Consume these types of fats instead of sweets, starches, and vegetable oils, which cause high blood sugar and weight gain. A recent study from Johns Hopkins University suggests that a low-carb, high-fat diet may be best for healthy weight loss. Just make sure those fats don't come from junk food.

7. **Pill popping**. Often, when weight loss gets tough, it's tempting to turn to one of the many pills, capsules, and powders that promise to reduce appetite cravings or increase fat or carbohydrate burning. Unfortunately these pills give you only a small increase in fat burning (see the QuickAndDirty-Tips.com article "Do Weight Loss Supplements Work?"). Also, people who rely on pills for weight loss are far less likely to engage in exercise and healthy eating, which get more significant results.

8. **Snacking**. In point 2, I emphasized that a high caloric intake, with the goal of sustaining the metabolism, often re-

sults in overeating. The same can be said for snacking. Flaxseed crackers, raw almonds, morning muesli, raw fruit, and cheese sticks often add up to an extra several hundred calories each day. Remember, covert calories add up quickly.

9. **Hormonal imbalances**. In the QuickandDirtyTips.com article "What Causes Cellulite," you learn that hormonal imbalances can be a prime cause of cellulite formation, particularly in women who are estrogen dominant. If you've tried everything to lose weight but have never had the levels of your estrogen, testosterone, or thyroid hormones tested, a hormonal imbalance may be is the cause of your inability to lose weight. Just be sure to get your blood tested by a doctor before adding supplements and medications to address a suspected issue.

10. **Food intolerances or allergies**. Bloating, weight gain, chronic fatigue, nutrient depletion, and an inability to exercise can all be related to eating foods your body is allergic to or simply doesn't have the enzymes to digest. Common triggers are wheat, soy, dairy, eggs, and fructose. A gluten-free diet may be one good place to start, but you should also consider getting tested for food allergies, using an elimination diet, introducing digestive enzymes, and keeping a food log. Always consult your doctor prior to drastically changing your diet or if you suspect an allergy.

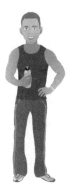

How to Measure Your Body Fat

In this section, you'll learn six ways to measure your body fat and why you should measure it in the first place.

What Is Body-Fat Percentage?

There are two different types of body fat. The first, your essential fat, is necessary for you to stay alive; essential fat levels are about 3 to 5 percent in men and 8 to 12 percent in women. When I was a bodybuilder, my total body fat dropped down to 2 percent, which meant my essential fat was very low, and I experienced mood swings, joint pain, and a loss of sex drive and appetite—along with other issues that correlate to a low essential body fat. Needless to say, as soon as I was done bodybuilding I got my hands on some ice cream and brought myself back up to a healthy body-fat level.

The second type of body fat is your storage fat, which is also known as adipose tissue. Some storage fat protects your organs or provides insulation, but for many people, it's just annoying energy waiting to be burned.

Why Measure Body Fat?

If you know your body-fat levels, then you have a number that you can use as a goal. For example, if you use any of the information in this article to find that your body-fat percentage is 30 percent, and your weight is 170 pounds, then you can calculate that 30 percent of 170 pounds is 51 pounds, and learn that's how many pounds of fat you have on your body. You can then make a goal to lose 10 pounds of fat in 5 weeks. If you don't lose any muscle along the way, then you'd weight 160 pounds, you'd have 41 pounds of body fat $(51 - 10 = 41)$ and your new body-fat percentage would be 25 percent.

But what if you do gain muscle? If you're just tracking your body weight, then you may be disappointed because the scale might not show that you're losing, even though your body-fat levels are going down. By using a body fat scale, you can track what is happening with your body fat even if your weight is not changing. Since muscle takes up far less space than fat, a gain in lean muscle accompanied by a loss in body fat can result in a smaller waistline, a flatter stomach, and a decrease in clothing size!

How to Measure Body Fat

Now that you know what body-fat percentage is and why you should measure it, here are six ways you can check your body fat:

1. **Underwater weighing (hydrodensitometry).** This option is usually offered at a university or laboratory. As the name implies, you are literally dunked underwater. While underwater, you let all the air out of your lungs and your body density is calculated. Body density can then be used to calculate body fat. Underwater weighing is considered the gold-standard measurement and is very accurate, but let's face it: unless winning money at the fair is involved, who wants to strip to his skivvies and get dunked in a big tub of water?

2. **Calipers.** Also known as the pinch method, a skinfold caliper measurement involves pinching and measuring the fat under your skin on three to seven different places on your body, and then using the thickness of these pinches of fat to calculate body fat percentage. Since it's quick and convenient, personal trainers at gyms often use these measurements. Unfortunately, unless you do many, many measurements, it is easy to vastly over- or underestimate the measurement, especially in overweight or obese individuals. If you use this method, ask the person measuring you how many times he or she has done caliper testing.

3. **DEXA.** DEXA, which stands for dual energy X-ray absorptiometry, is a full body scan commonly used to measure bone density that can also be used to measure body fat and show

exactly where the fat is distributed. This is one of the more costly methods of measurement and is probably not an option for people who like to avoid X-ray radiation; but if you're been diagnosed with a chronic disease related to obesity or overweight, you may be able to get your health insurance to cover the cost. Though less common than DEXA, other full body scanning devices that can measure body fat include magnetic resonance imaging (MRI), total body electrical conductivity (TOBEC), and computed tomography (CT scan).

4. **NIR**. In NIR (near infrared interactance), a fiber-optic probe is held against your skin (usually against your biceps), a light is used to penetrate the tissues, and the light is then reflected off your bones back into the detector, which approximates your body fat based on a prediction equation that also takes into consideration your height, weight, body type, and level of activity. Although simple and noninvasive, this method can have a high degree of error in people with high or low body-fat percentages, and it also requires an experienced technician. Your level of hydration and skin color can also affect the accuracy of this measurement.

5. **BodPod**. A space-age-looking pod that can be found at many fancier health clubs, the BodPod uses sensors to measure how much air your body displaces while you sit inside the small chamber. This information is then used to determine your body density and then estimate your body fat.

6. **BIA**. Somewhat similar to NIR, BIA, which stands for bioelectrical impedance analysis, involves sending a painless electrical signal into your body; this signal passes through fat, muscle, and water at different speeds. The speed of the

signal's passing is then combined with your sex, height, weight, and activity levels to approximate your body-fat percentage. Once again, if you're dehydrated, overhydrated, or skinny or overweight, this measurement can be inaccurate— but it is commonly used in body-fat scales or handheld devices because it is relatively inexpensive and portable.

Finally, at the time this book was going to press, I learned about another extremely accurate ultrasound measuring device for tracking body fat. You can learn more about it in podcast episode #170 from BenGreenfieldFitness.com.

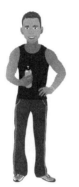

10 Tips to Build Muscle Fast

Whether you want to bulk up, get more curvaceous calves, enhance your chest, or achieve any other muscle-building goal, you're about to get ten tips to build muscle fast. If you combine these tips with the workouts you find in this book, you'll literally see your body morph as you add lean muscle!

1. **Lift**. The only way to significantly increase muscle is to cause muscle fibers to tear, and the only way to do that is to subject your muscles to external forces to which they're not accustomed. So unless you have a heavy manual labor job like moving or construction, you must get your hands on barbells, dumbbells, and weight lifting machines to see significant progress in muscle building.

2. **Go multi-joint**. Unless you're already very muscular, single-joint movements such as biceps curls or triceps extensions

do not build muscle quickly. Instead, you should use multi-joint exercises such as cleans, dead lifts, squats, and bench pressing. Not only do these exercises work more muscles in less time, but they also allow you to use much heavier weight than you can lift with single-joint exercises.

3. **Go heavy**. Most people who are trying to build muscle do not use heavy enough weight. You should be lifting in the range of 8–12 repetitions per set, performing 3–8 sets per exercise, and using a weight that leads to muscle failure by the end of each set. One of the reasons that bodybuilders exercise with a partner is so that someone is there to help them when the weight gets too heavy to lift with good form. If you don't have a workout partner, you can simply stop when you get too tired to lift with good form, rest a few seconds, then keep lifting to complete the set. This is a better way to build muscle than using a weight that allows you to comfortably complete a set without reaching muscle failure.

4. **Avoid cardio**. Your body requires calories to build muscle, and if you are doing a significant amount of cardio exercise like running or bicycling, you are burning calories that your body could otherwise be using to build muscle. So if you want to build muscle as quickly as possible, only use cardio for a brief warm-up and then focus on weight training.

5. **Eat**. To put on one pound of muscle, you need to consume at least 3,500 extra calories. Since an achievable rate of muscle gain is 1–2 pounds per week, you will need to be eating 500–1,000 extra calories per day to get 3,500–7,000 extra calories each week. But rather than indiscriminately shoving food down the hatch, try to consume calories from healthy protein sources (grass-fed beef), healthy fat sources (avocados

and coconut milk), and healthy carbohydrate sources (sweet potatoes).

6. **Supplement**. In the article "Do Muscle Building Supplements Work?" at QuickandDirtyTips.com, I reviewed several popular muscle-building supplements. The top two most effective supplements you should be consuming to gain muscle quickly are a high quality protein powder and a creatine supplement. Other popular muscle-building supplements, such as nitric oxide or beta-alanine, will achieve small results, but for your money will not be as effective as the legal protein and creatine supplements.

7. **Rest**. If you work a muscle too hard too many days in a row, the muscle fibers will become too damaged to properly repair and grow. To build muscle quickly, you must completely fatigue a muscle group, but then give it time to rest. Typically, a muscle needs at least 72 hours to properly repair from a muscle-building weight training session. A good rule to follow is to allow for complete absence of soreness in a muscle before working that muscle again. For example, do a shoulders and chest workout on Monday and Thursday, a leg workout on Tuesday and Friday, and a back, arms, and abs workout on Wednesday and Saturday.

8. **Recover**. While you are resting, be sure to give your body what it needs to properly recover and put the muscles into a state of optimal growth. Activities that enhance recovery include ice baths or cold showers, compression clothing, massage therapy or foam rolling, stretching, breathing exercises, and adequate sleep.

9. **Destress**. High levels of stress can quickly drain testosterone, an anabolic muscle-building hormone, and increase

levels of cortisol, a catabolic muscle-damaging hormone. If you find yourself constantly cranky or with a fast heart rate at work or school, it's likely that you're too stressed for optimal muscle growth. Teach yourself to relax, breathe deeply, and plan out your day to give yourself more time and less stress.

10. **Address Hormones**. If you are above the age of thirty, hormonal deficiencies can slow your rate of muscle gain. If you feel your muscle gain is too slow, consider going to a doctor to test your hormone levels and address any imbalances or deficiencies.

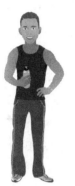

10 Tips for Proper Gym Etiquette

I was recently talking to a gym-goer who said that he was all fired up about a guy at the gym who took weights off the dumbbell rack and proceeded to do shoulder raises directly in front of the mirror, blocking everyone else's access to the dumbbell rack.

Was he right or wrong to be upset about this? Is there indeed proper gym etiquette?

As a matter of fact, there actually is gym etiquette, but it's often not written down anywhere. So here are ten quick and dirty tips for how to behave at the gym.

1. **Wipe up after yourself**. Most gyms have towels available at the front desk or somewhere near the exercise equipment. These towels are not there just in case you spill a big cup of soda or need to teasingly towel-whip a workout buddy. They

are there so that you can wipe annoying sweat from your body and mop up any nasty, stinky wet puddles on the exercise equipment or floor. If your gym doesn't have towels, then bring your own or just use an old T-shirt. And yes, when you wipe up sweat, you are expected to use disinfectant spray if your gym has provided it or made it readily accessible in the workout area.

2. **It's okay to spot and be spotted**. Often, when lifting heavy weights, you or another exerciser may need a spot, which is assistance or a helpful hand while you are performing the exercise. If there are no personal trainers or gym employees available to help you, it is okay to ask someone else for help provided that

- You are 100 percent confident that the person has the physical capability to help you.
- You understand if he or she says no.
- You do not interrupt another person's exercise routine to ask. In other words, if you are about to attempt a new personal record bench press, do not go tap a scrawny teenager on the shoulder as he is deeply involved in an exercise, headphones attached.

    Similarly, if someone asks you for help, it is fine to politely decline if

- You do not feel physically capable.
- You are busy with your own exercise routine.
- A personal trainer or gym employee is available in the workout area.

3. **Give others space**. Often dumbbells, barbells, and other pieces of equipment are on racks or shelves. When you re-

trieve of these items from its location, back at least 4 to 6 feet away so that others can easily access the equipment while you're doing your exercise. If there is absolutely no way to do this, then go find the owner of your gym and tell him or her to read this article, because owners are legally required to include a minimum of 3 feet of space between equipment and enough room to perform exercises without impeding gym traffic.

4. **Leave it how you found it, usually.** If you are using weight machines or equipment that has weight stacks or special settings and you are not completely sure whether someone else was using the equipment or is in the process of using the equipment, then you must leave it how you found it. If nobody appears to be using it, you can change the adjustments and do your sets or your exercises, but once you are finished, restore it to how you found it. This means that you should return the stack to its original weight and the height of the seat to its original setting unless you are 100 percent confident that nobody else is in the process of using the equipment.

5. **Have good hygiene.** Nobody likes to smell cigarette residue, heavy body odor, or stinky farts while exercising. Please shower or use deodorant prior to exercising in public areas. If you need to break wind, politely enter the restroom, do your business, and then continue with your workout. If your exercise session includes a pool or a post-workout soak in the hot tub, you must shower beforehand with soap. When it comes to gym etiquette, Pig-Pen is not a good role model.

6. **Clean up after yourself.** You've already learned that you need to wipe up your sweat. You also need to be sure to

remove hats, towels, sports drinks, or any other clutter from equipment that you're done using. You also need to pick up wrappers, crumbs, or sauces from any food that you have consumed during your workout (if you are lucky enough to be working out at a gym that even allows you to eat in the workout area, which most gyms do not).

7. **Don't monopolize equipment**. If you are using a piece of cardio equipment or a weight machine and you need to use the restroom, do a quick burst of cardio or mix in a set on one other piece of equipment, then leave a hat, towel, or other sign that you are temporarily reserving that piece of equipment. However, if someone is obviously waiting to use the equipment or you plan on being gone longer than a couple of minutes, then do not reserve or attempt to monopolize the machine.

   You'll simply need to share and let someone else work in a set along with you, which means you'll also need to wipe down that piece of equipment after each set that you do. In the same manner, if you want to use a piece of equipment that someone appears to be using for an unreasonably long period of time, politely ask whether you can share that area with them. If they say no, then trust me, it's not worth the fight; although you can, if you really want to, approach a personal trainer or gym employee to voice your complaint.

8. **Read the clothing rules or ask**. Guys, in most cases, nobody really wants to see your nipples or copious amounts of chest and back hair at the gym. And ladies, unless you are thoroughly confident that nobody at the gym will complain about your butt hanging out of your gym shorts, wear

something that keeps your body parts relatively contained. Most gyms post basic clothing rules, which are typically:

- Wear a shirt.
- Wear closed-toe shoes.
- Don't wear jeans (they can destroy the vinyl on the equipment).
- If you have a baby, make sure he or she has an appropriate waterproof diaper in the pool.

In most cases, it's best to err on the safe side and not wear clothing that you suspect may offend or nauseate others.

9. **Use sign-up forms properly**. If you have reserved a treadmill or bicycle or if you have signed up for a class, then cross out your name from the sign-in list if you decide not to use the equipment or attend the class. If a class is full and you want to attend, it's okay to just drop in and ask the instructor, since there are often no-shows.

10. **Don't try to solve conflicts yourself**. If a fellow gym-goer appears to be breaking any of these rules, do not attempt to resolve the conflict yourself. In almost every case, the appropriate step is to locate a personal trainer or gym employee and allow him or her to mediate the situation. People can get aggressive, grumpy, and downright mean when they're exercising, and the last thing you need at the gym is a bloody nose. That's not what those towels are for.

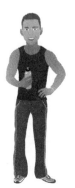

17 Gym Terms You Need to Know

Fitting in at the gym can go beyond simply being polite; you have to know the lingo if you really want to fit in. So in this section, you'll learn seventeen common gym terms, from gym equipment to exercise movements to common gym phrases, and how to understand workout instructions or conversations that you hear or take part in at the gym.

Gym Equipment Lingo

Let's begin with some of the common equipment you'll find lying around the gym.

Barbell ✧ This is a long bar that typically weights 35–45 pounds, although there are lighter versions at most commercial gyms. You load weight on both ends of a barbell to increase the resistance. Don't let your ego get in the way when using a barbell—it's easy to get injured with these.

Cables ✧ A cable exercise apparatus is typically comprised of some type of handle, like a rope or bar, attached to a pulley via a cable, which is then attached to a stack of weights. By using the combination of handle, pulley, and cable, you can manipulate large amounts of weight and move in many different ranges of motion that would be difficult or impossible with a barbell or dumbbell.

Dumbbell ✧ Dumbbells are typically comprised of a handle between two weights. They can be used individually or two at the same time. Dumbbells can be adjustable, meaning you can add resistance by attaching more weight to the dumbbell, or fixed, meaning that you can't change the weight.

Dumbbells are highly versatile and can be used for a wide range of exercises. You'll typically find them stored on a sturdy shelf called a rack. Be careful the dumbbells don't fall off the rack or your toes could pay a hefty price!

Free Weights ✧ If it's designed for exercise and not attached to some kind of pulley or machine, you can call it a free weight. This term covers barbells, dumbbells, medicine balls, kettlebells, or anything else you can grab and do a variety of exercises with, assuming it's not a small, defenseless person. Free weights are good to include in your program because they use many stabilizing and balancing muscles.

Plate ✧ Plates are the weights that go on each end of a barbell or adjustable dumbbell. In America, plates typically weigh 45, 35, 25, 10, 5, or 2.5 pounds, while most international plates are 25, 20, 17, 10, 5, 2.5, 2, or 1 kilogram.

Smith Machine ✧ This machine, named after a gym owner who invented it, is comprised of a barbell that moves in a stationary track, which ensures that the barbell moves only vertically and in a controlled path. It can be used when you need to press or lift heavy weights with a barbell, but don't have someone to help you.

Stack ◊ On a weight lifting machine or cable apparatus, the resistance is provided by a stack, which is usually several rectangular plates stacked on top of one another. Resistance can then selected by using a pin that can be placed at a chosen place on the stack. Interestingly, a stack can also refer to taking several nutritional supplements at once.

Exercise Lingo

Here are some terms you may come across in workout instructions, exercise books, and fitness magazines.

Recovery ◊ When you perform an exercise, you'll eventually get to the point where you need a specified number of seconds or minutes to rest or go easy. That is referred to as your recovery period, and typically varies from 30 seconds up to several minutes.

Reps ◊ The word *reps* is short for repetitions and means the number of times you perform an exercise movement, which typically ranges from 3 up to 30, depending on the type of workout you're doing.

Set ◊ A set is a group of repetitions, and typically you will perform 2 to 8 or more sets for any given exercise. For example, if you are trying to get a toned butt, you might do 5 sets of 12 reps of a reverse lunge exercise.

Spin ◊ Contrary to popular belief, this is not some type of indoor craft class, but is actually a form of cycling that is performed on a special bike called a spin bike, and usually occurs in a group training environment. Typically spin bikes have a wheel called a flywheel that provides the resistance, so they're a bit different from a regular stationary bicycle.

Tempo ✧ Many workout books, magazines, or programs now indicate tempo, which simply refers to the speed at which you lift. For example, if you take 3 seconds to lift a weight, hold the weight for 1 second at the top of the movement, then take 2 seconds to lower the weight, the tempo would be 3:1:2.

Common Gym Phrases

Finally, you may hear the following phrases pop up in conversations at the gym.

Failure ✧ Rather than indicating that you did a bad job at something, the term *failure*, when used in an exercise environment, simply means that you got to the point of physical exhaustion, which often occurs in sets designed to build muscle.

Max ✧ This term is short for the maximum amount of weight one is able to lift in a specific exercise. It is safe to assume that someone who frequently uses this term may not be telling the entire truth.

Spot ✧ People may ask you if they can get a spot; they are not asking for you for help in finding their dog. Instead they are asking you to help them do an exercise with a weight they probably can't lift themselves.

PR or PB ✧ Short for personal record or personal best, this is used to describe a new personal achievement, such as running 3 miles in 20 minutes, being able to bench press 200 pounds, or sticking to a New Year's resolution for longer than 10 days.

Work In ✧ If someone asks you to work in, this means he or she would like to share a piece of equipment at the gym with you, perhaps by alternating sets on an exercise machine or by using dumbbells that you're doing sets with.

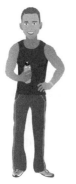

Techniques to Get Better Results from Weight Lifting

SAID, or specific adaptations to imposed demands, is a principle in exercise. It means that our bodies eventually adapt to the demands we place upon them. For people who lift weights, that means you must constantly change or alter your routine in some way in order to burn more calories, make your weight lifting workouts harder, and get better results.

But there is far more you can do to make a weight lifting workout harder than simply adding more weight. So here are ten quick and dirty tips for getting more work done, burning more calories, and making your muscles feel it more.

1. **Bouncing**. Rather than taking a pogo stick to the gym, bouncing actually involves doing mini-reps at end ROM. Yes, that last bit of lingo may require some explaining. ROM stands for range of motion, and end ROM refers to the very

end of the range of motion. For example, the end ROM of a body weight squat is when your knees are bent, at the very bottom of the motion. At this point in the squat, you could do 5–10 mini-reps, or very short, bouncy squats, and then stand. Bouncing works for push-ups, crunches, lunges, curls, and just about any basic movement.

2. **Explosions**. Pyromaniac readers, please settle down—this has nothing to do with dynamite. For explosions, hold a movement in the toughest position, then explode quickly up and down, then back into toughest position. For example, when you get to the bottom of a push-up, you can hold for 1–2 seconds, then push up as fast as possibly (your hands can even leave the ground) and land back in the bottom of the push-up.

3. **Quarter reps**. For quarter reps, you do your exercise normally, but in the very middle of the movement you stop, do a quarter rep, and then continue. For example, while performing a lunge you would stop when your knee is halfway bent, stand halfway, then continue through the lunge, which basically turns every 1 rep into 1.5 reps.

4. **Ladder reps**. For ladder reps, do 5 mini-reps in the bottom range of motion, 5 mini-reps in the middle range of motion, and 5 mini-reps in the top range of motion. For example, during a triceps body weight dip, you would do 5 reps with your elbows bent at the bottom of the dip, 5 reps in the middle of the dip, and then 5 reps at the top of the dip.

5. **Stripping**. Contrary to how it might sound, stripping does not involve taking your clothes off at the gym (although pole dancing cardio classes are increasing in popularity). Instead, stripping involves lifting a weight until you cannot

perform any more repetitions, decreasing (or stripping) the weight, then continuing with the same exercise for as many repetitions as possible. In a single set, you can strip the weight to your heart's content, until an embarrassingly small weight is making you grunt and groan.

6. **Supersets**. In a superset, you perform an exercise set immediately after a different exercise set, with no rest in between. There are three different types of supersets.

   In the first, you do a set for one muscle group, such as leg extensions for your quadriceps, then with no rest, do a set for the opposing muscle group, such as leg curls for your hamstrings.

   In the second, you perform both sets for the same muscle group, such as chest flies followed by chest presses.

   Finally, you can do a giant superset, in which you perform three to four back-to-back exercises for the same muscle group, such as triceps pushdowns to narrow grip push-ups to dips to triceps overhead extensions.

7. **Super slow sets**. As you might guess, in a super slow set, you perform your repetitions in a slow controlled manner. Though super slow training can be a waste of time to do all the time, if something like a regular push-up is very easy for you, try to do a push-up with a four-count down and a four-count back up. See what I mean?

8. **Forced repetitions**. Forced repetitions are exercises assisted by a training partner, or spotter. These are typically performed with a much heavier weight than you could normally lift on your own, or involve significantly more repetitions than you could do by yourself. As you reach failure, your spotter helps you, or forces you, to complete the set.

9. **Negatives**. In a negative set, you slowly lower a weight heavier than one you would normally use, and either cheat to raise the weight back up or have a partner help you. For example, if you are trying to increase the amount of weight you can bench press, you would slowly lower a heavy weight to your chest, then have a spotter grab the bar and assist you in pushing the weight back up to the starting position.

10. **Cheating**. Speaking of cheating, believe it or not, this is actually another strategy. Although attention to good form is usually recommended when you are lifting weights, cheating may involve rocking back and forth with your body, arching your back, or using an extra part of your body to perform an exercise. For example, if you are pressing a weight overhead with one arm, you may jump, arch, or use the opposing arm to help you out just a bit.

Now that you know how to bounce, explode, cheat, and strip, you have no excuse not to get more results from your weight lifting.

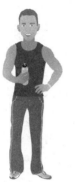

10 Exercise Motivation Tips

Motivating yourself to get fit goes above and beyond simply throwing some upbeat music into your audio player! Here are ten more exercise motivation tips.

1. **Try caffeine**. Beyond simply stimulating your central nervous system to release energy-bestowing adrenaline, caffeine can make working out seem less hard, which is also known as reducing your rating of perceived exertion. A cup of coffee 30–60 minutes before working out is one way to get your caffeine. Most popular weight-loss supplements also include this motivational drug.

2. **Clip pictures**. If there's a body or a look that you're trying to achieve—like a better butt, a flat stomach, or more shapely calves—then look for photos of that look in fitness magazines

or books. If you clip these pictures and keep them in a public place, such as on your refrigerator or bathroom mirror, or in a private spot like a diary or photo gallery on your phone, you'll have a constant reminder of why you're exercising.

3. **Use social accountability**. If you go on your Facebook page or the Facebook.com/GetFitGuy page or start a blog or a Twitter account, you can tell others about your exercise goals and your workout achievements. Social accountability and the ability to brag to others are great ways to get externally motivated to exercise.

4. **Get a workout buddy**. To keep you from sleeping through a workout, there's nothing like knowing a friend is tapping his or her feet waiting for you to show up for a early morning run. If you have trouble roping a friend into your fitness plans, check at your local gym for fitness groups or exercise clubs, like Masters' swim classes, triathlon training groups, or circuit training groups. And if you really want a fitness-specific friend, check out the next tip.

5. **Consider a personal trainer**. Though a friend can certainly motivate you to exercise, a personal trainer will push you, provide you with a plan, and get you workout results even faster. For help with finding a personal trainer, check out the QuickandDirtyTips.com article "How to Choose a Personal Trainer."

6. **Make a plan**. Even if you can't afford a personal trainer, plan the kind of workout you're going to do so that when you roll out of bed each morning, you've scheduled exercise in your daily routine. You can get plans from books, magazines, and Web sites. Some are free, but the better plans

typically cost a small amount—though still far less than the investment in a coach or trainer.

7. **Keep a Log**. By creating your planned workouts, then filling in a quick description of how you did or even simply checking off the workout as completed, you harness the power of the pen to keep you motivated to exercise. Motivation experts around the world have known for a long time that a key element in achieving any goal is to write it down!

8. **Take pictures**. You've already learned to collect pictures of the body that you want to achieve, but you also need to take pictures of yourself, especially if your goal is aesthetic, such as shedding fat or adding muscle. Try to take front and side pictures each week, with the same background and lighting. You'll be able to see results and use them to motivate yourself.

9. **The scale**. Yes, the dreaded scale can be a good exercise motivation tool, as can body-fat measurements, time-over-distance trials for riding a bike or running, or finding out how much you can bench press or squat. These are all examples of quantitative measurements, and though a photo can show you the quality of your progress, it takes some type of scale or number-based record keeping to show the quantity of your progress. And progress is motivating.

10. **Self-talk**. Never underestimate the importance of talking yourself up. From a simple self-motivating sentence such as "I can do this!" to an all-out furious and angry speech to yourself to keep you from skipping your trip to the gym on the drive home from work, the simple act of putting your workout goals and your workout excuses into words can get you to actually work out!

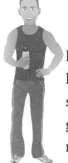

In addition to the exercise photos below (featuring me and my lovely wife Jessa), there is a growing database of exercise and stretching photos and videos at GetFitGuy.com/exercises, so go there if you are scratching your head on an exercise or want new moves!

Bodyweights

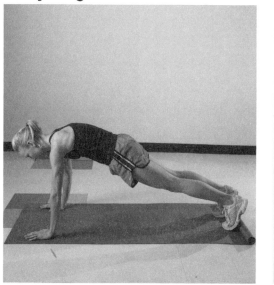
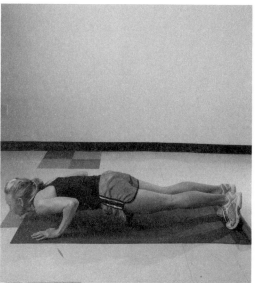

Push-up

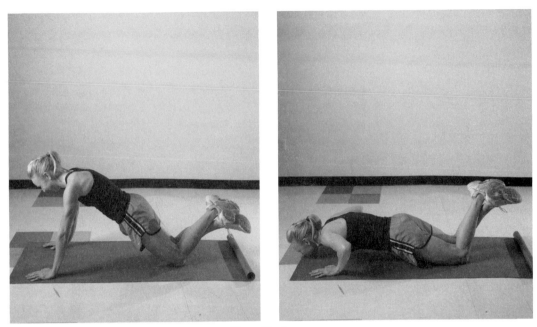

Knee Push-up

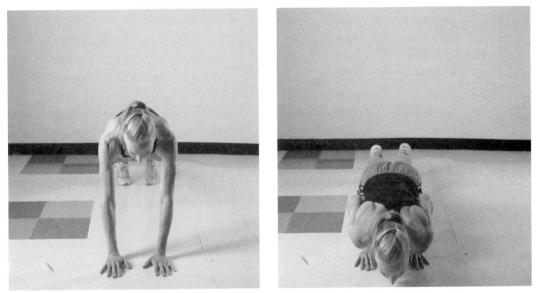

Narrow Grip Push-up

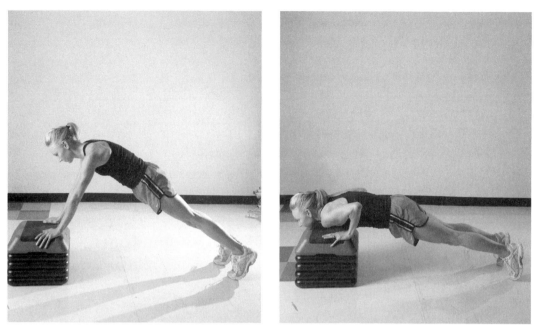

Incline Push-up

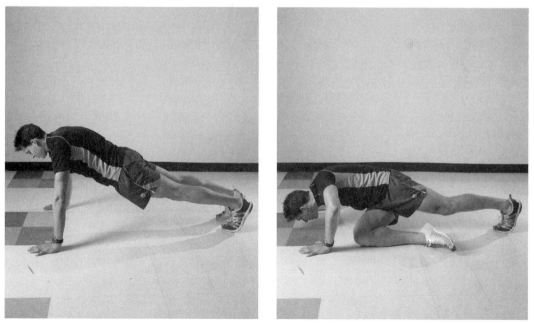

Spiderman Push-up

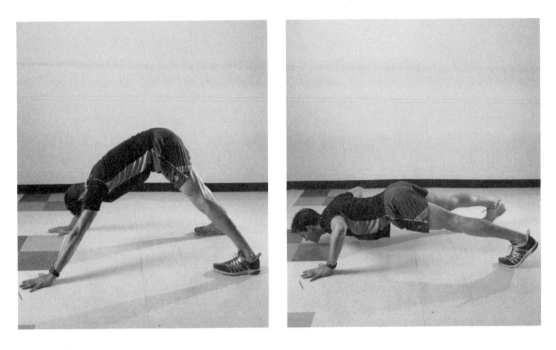

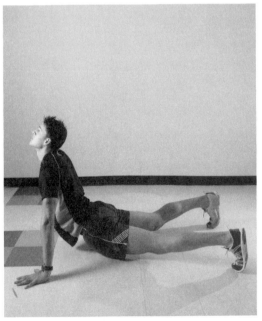

Dive Bomber Push-up

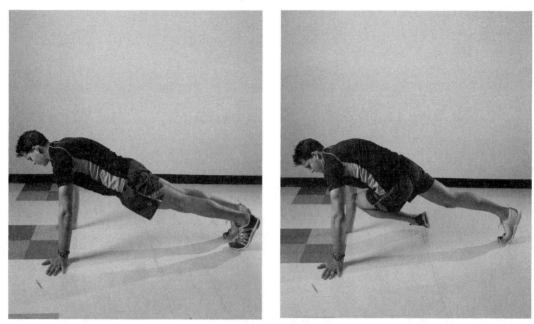

Mountain Climber

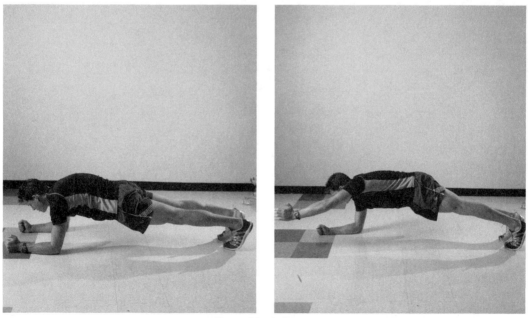

Front Plank Reach

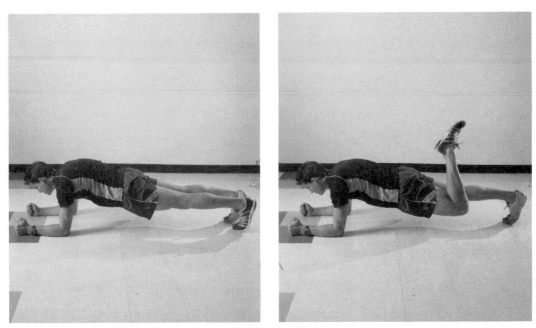

Front Plank Tap

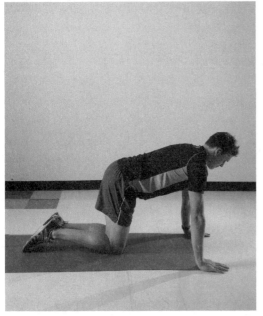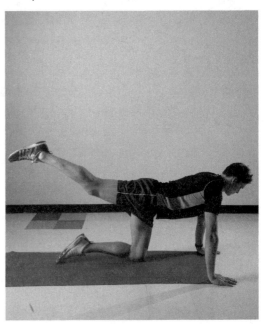

Kickout

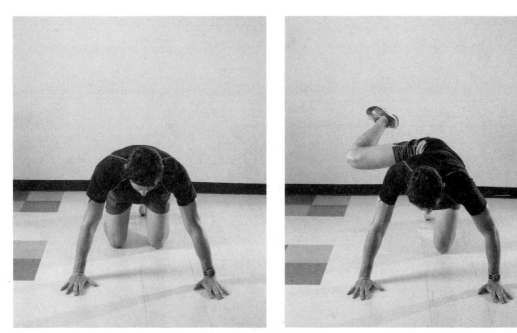

Fire Hydrant

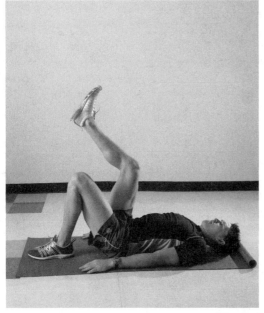 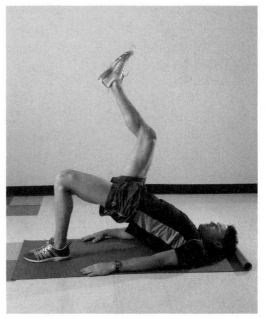

Single-Leg Bridge

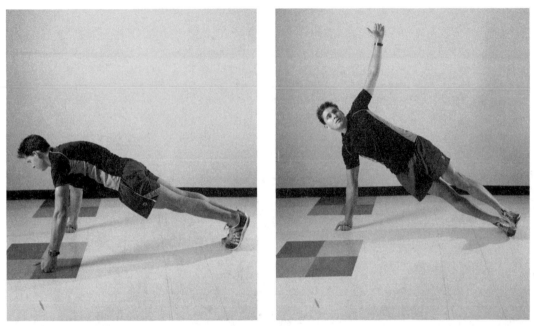

Corkscrew

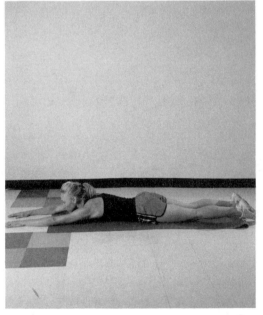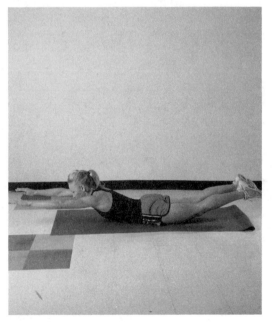

Superman

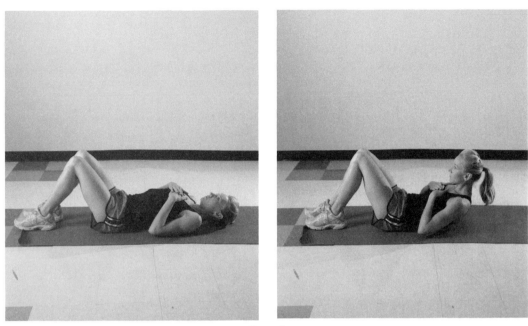

Crunch

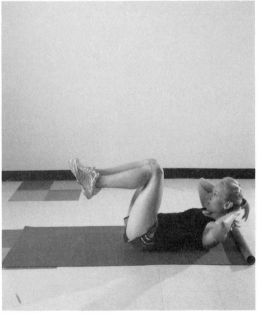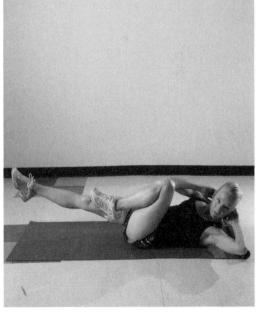

Bicycle Crunch

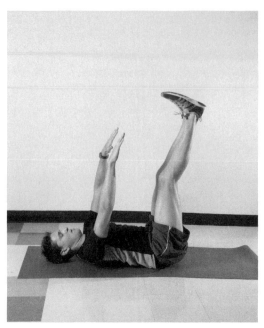 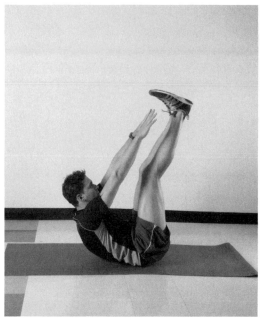

V Up

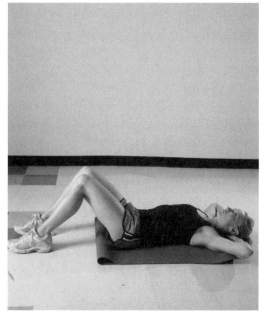 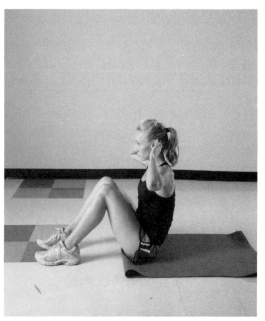

Sit-up

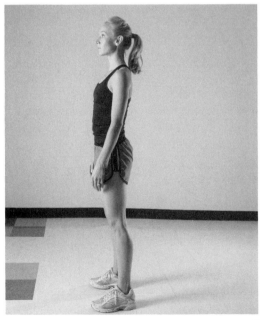

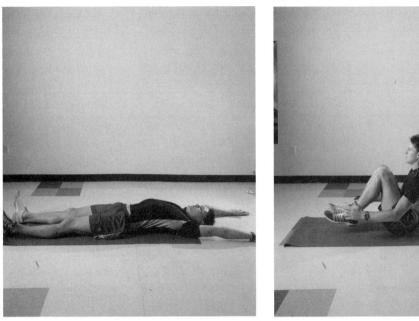

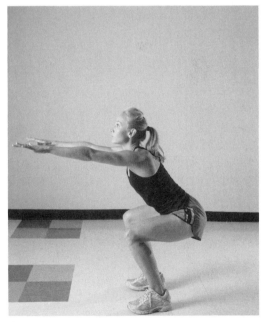

Little Big

Squat

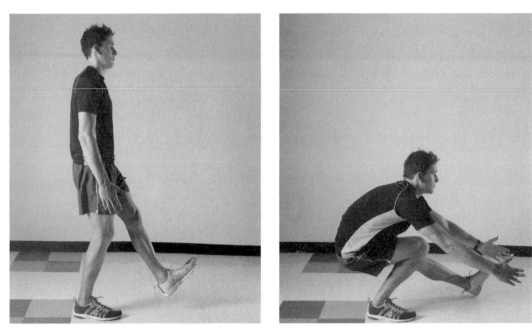

Single-Leg Squat

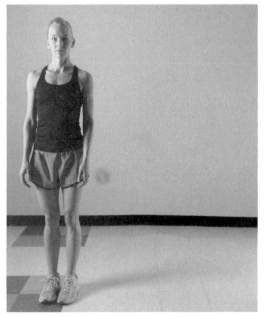
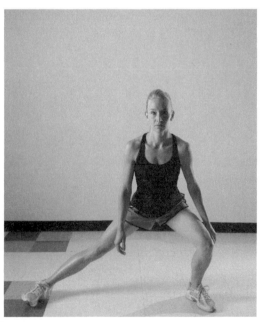

Lateral Lunge

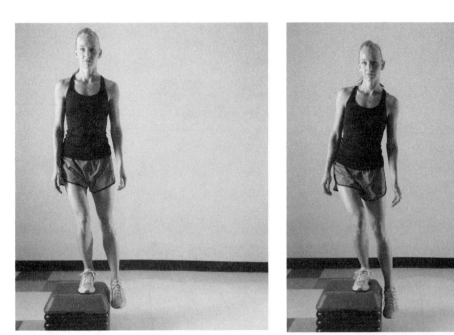

Hip Hike

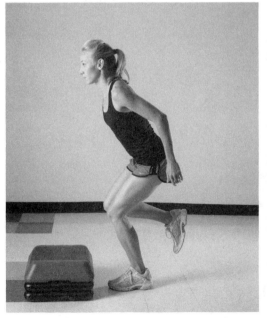
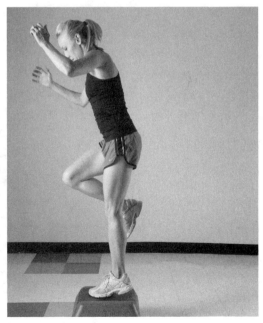

Single-Leg Hops

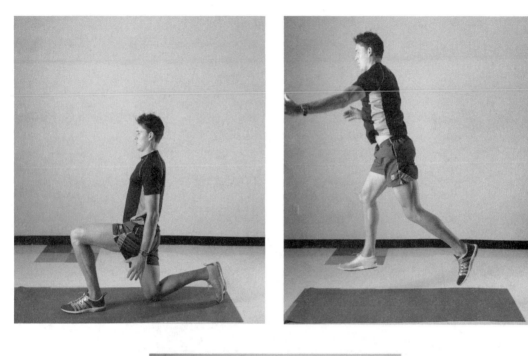

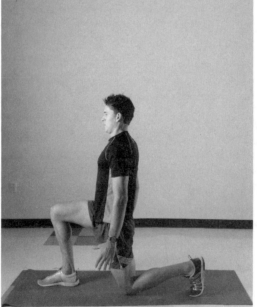

Lunge Jump

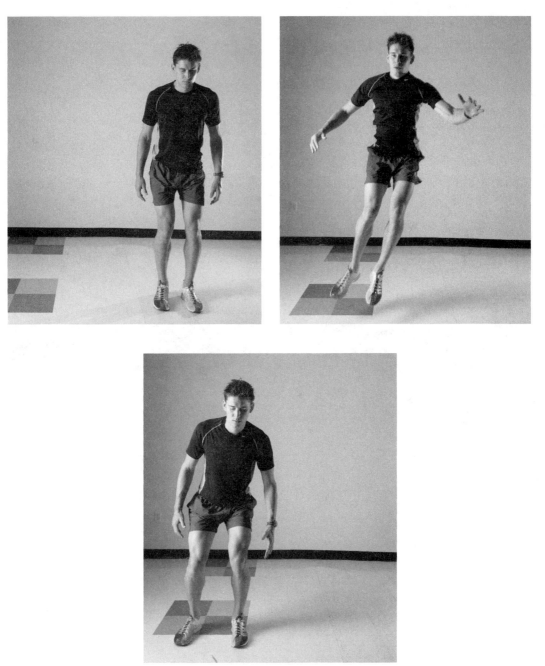

Side to Side Hops

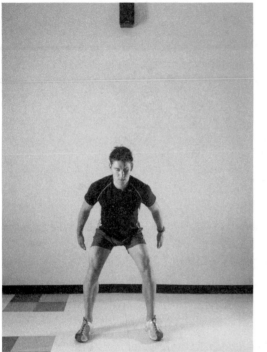 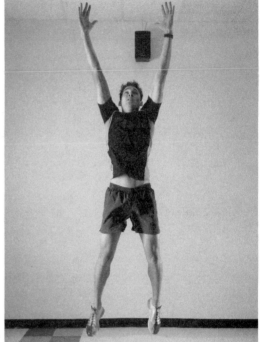

Vertical Jump

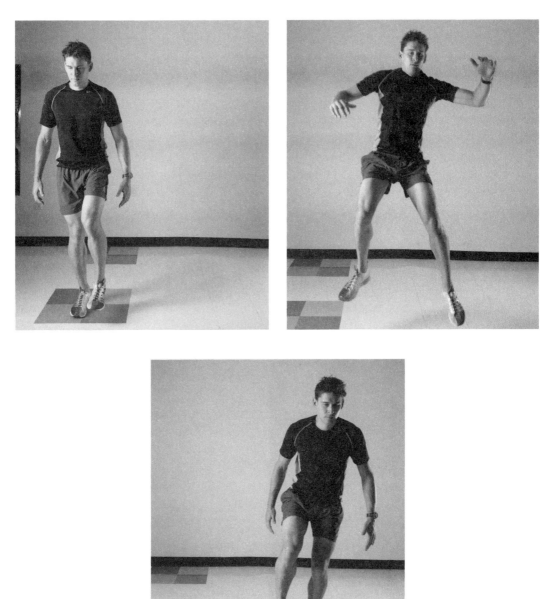

Skaters

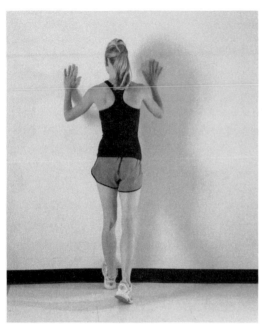

Wall Calf Stretch

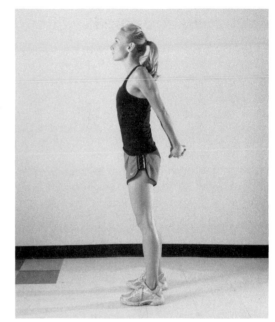

Anterior Shoulder Press

Dumbbells & Barbells

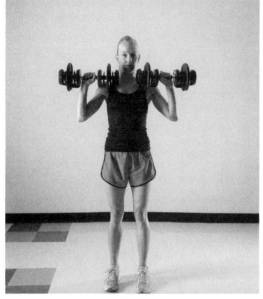
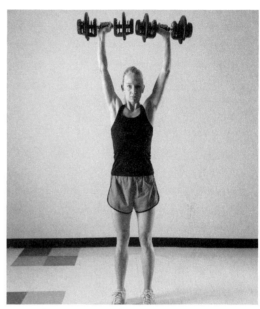

Dumbbell Overhead Press

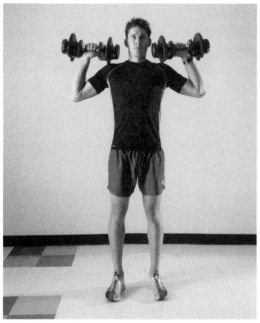
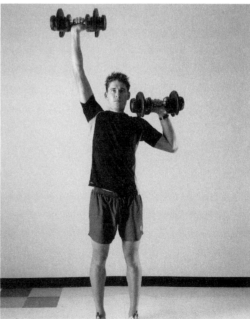

Alternating Overhead Press

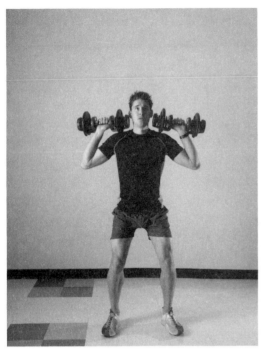
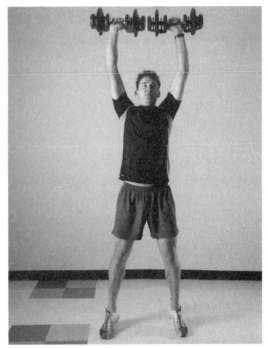

Overhead Push Press

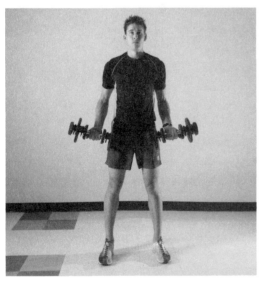
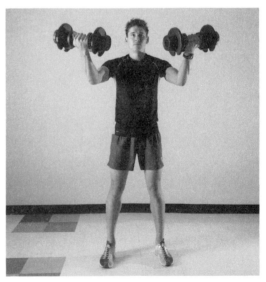

Uppercut

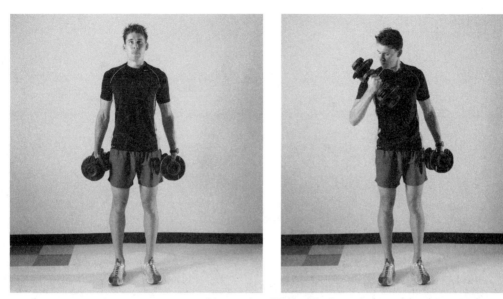

Alternating Biceps Curls

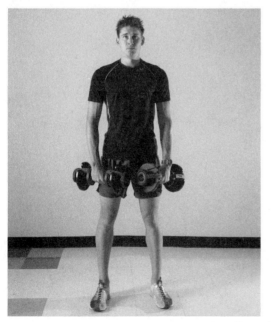 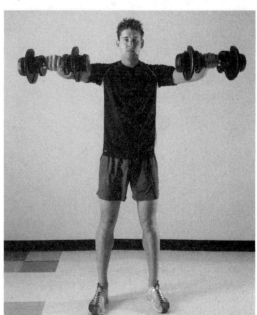

Front Raises

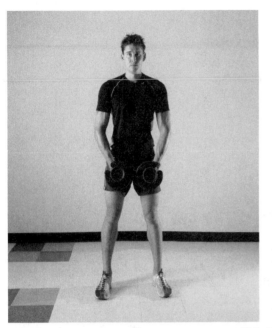 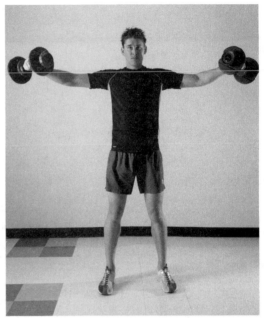

Side Raise

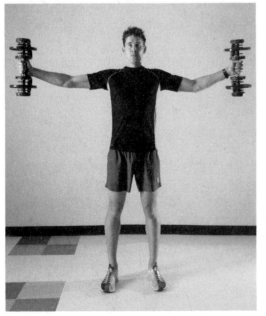 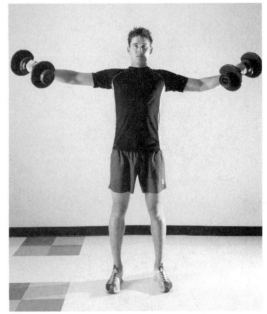

Empty Can

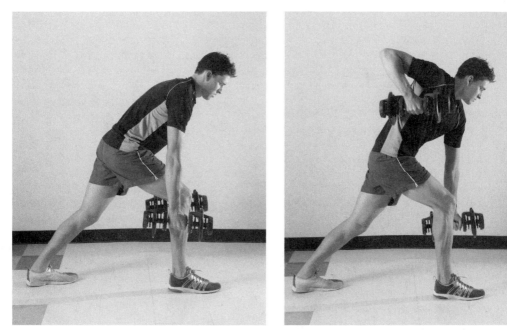

Alternating Bent Dumbbell Row Lunge

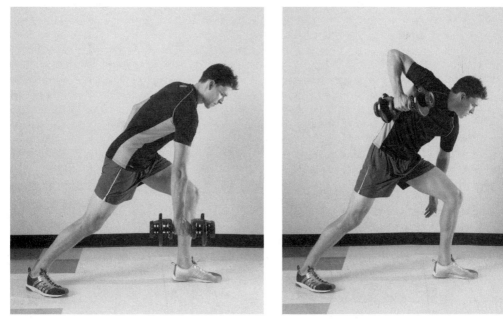

Single-Arm Dumbbell Row

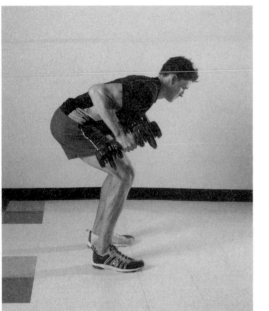
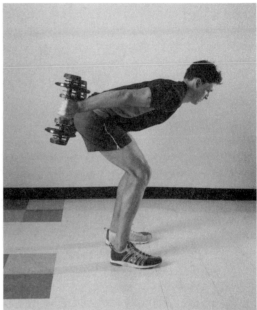

Dumbbell Kickbacks

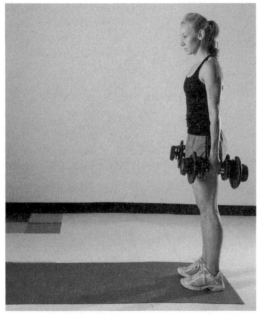
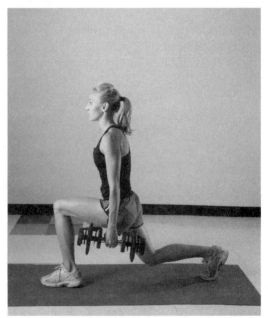

Lunge Step

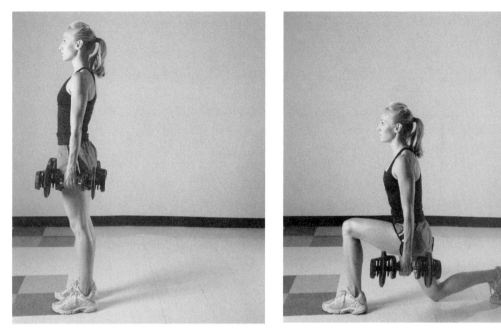

Reverse Lunge

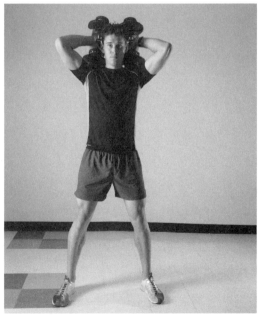

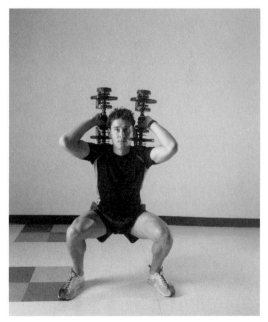

Dumbbell Squat

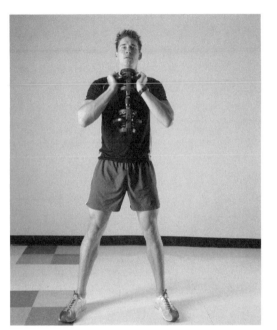
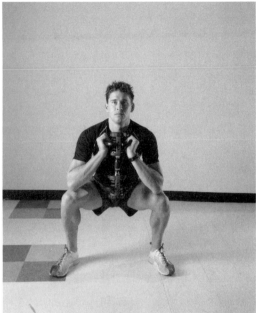

Goblet Squat

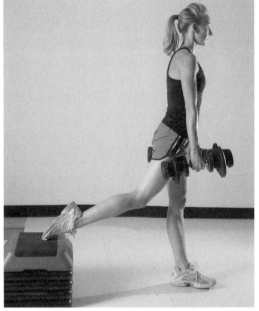
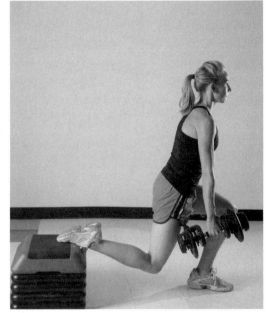

Split Squat

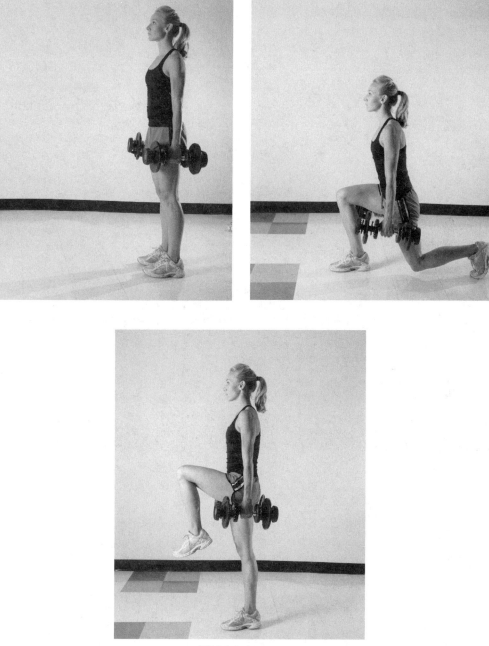

Walking Lunge

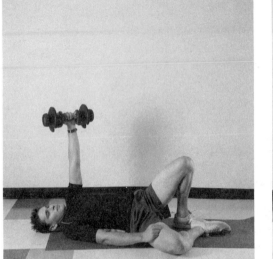
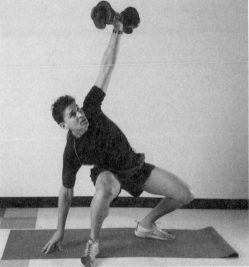

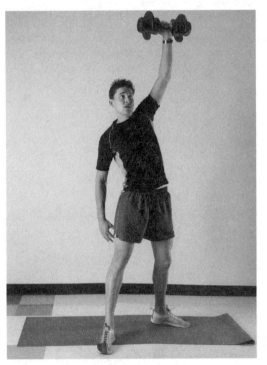

Turkish Get-up

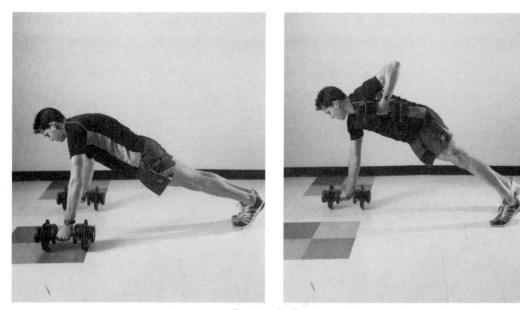

Renegade Row

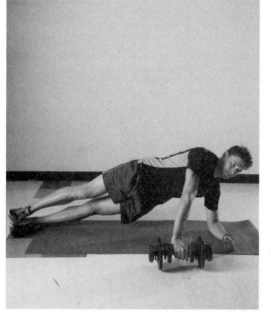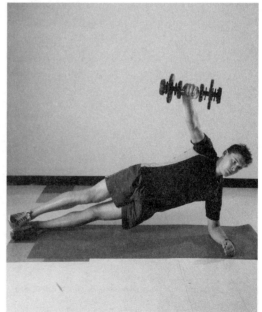

Side Plank Lateral Raise

Side Plank Rotation

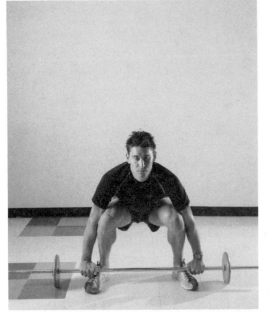
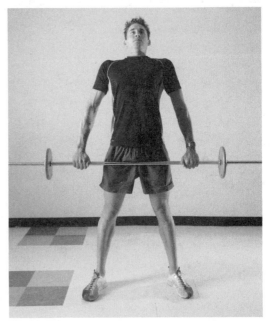

Dead Lift

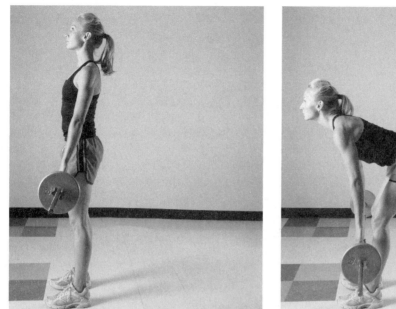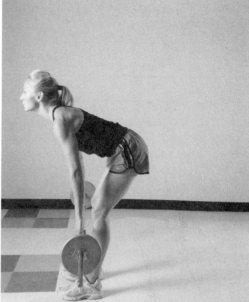

Romanian Dead Lift

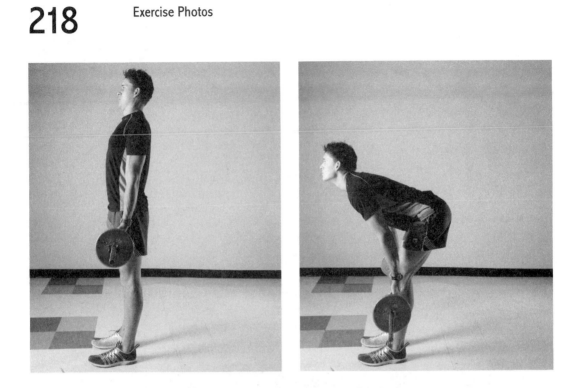

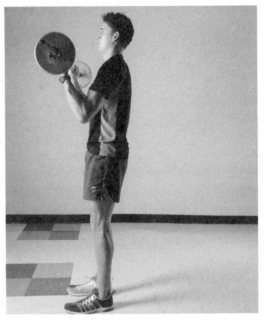

Romanian Dead Lift to Biceps Curl

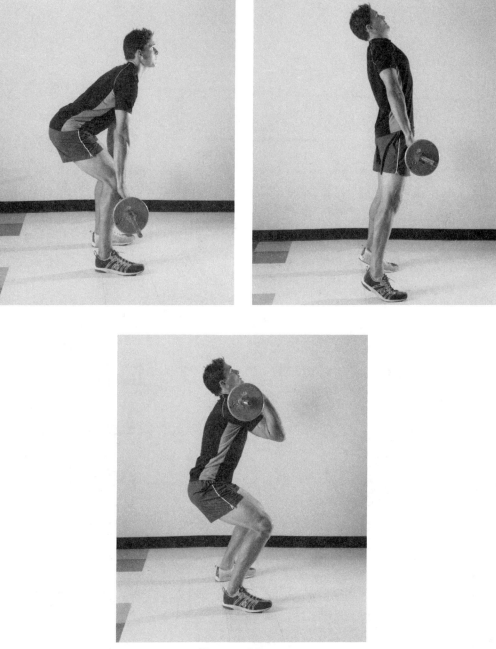

Clean and Press

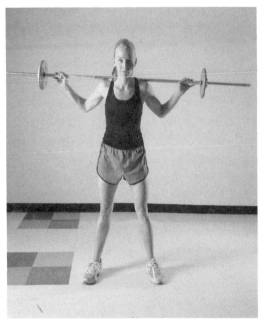 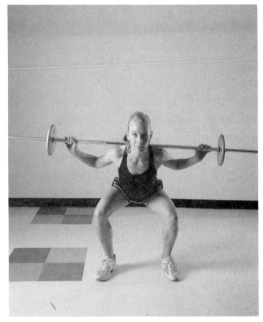

Barbell Squat

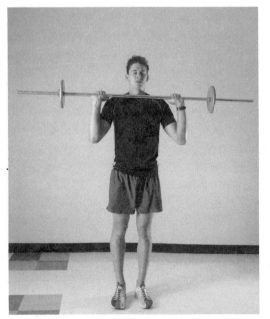 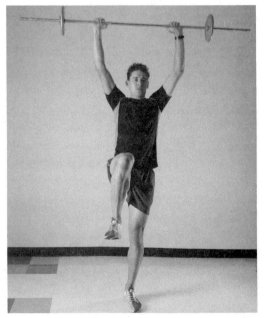

Single-Leg Overhead Press with Knee Drive

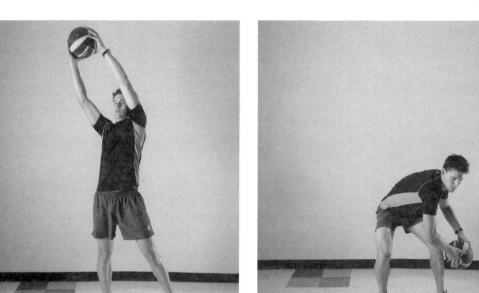

Medicine Ball Woodchopper

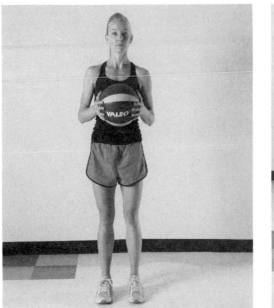

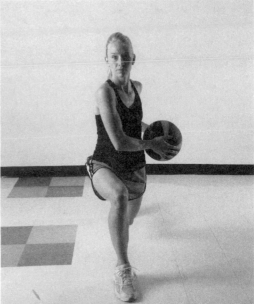

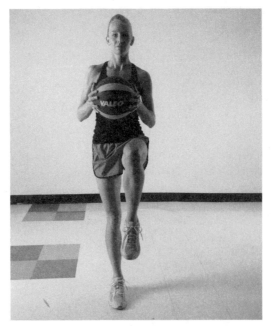

Walking Lunge with Twist

Stability Ball

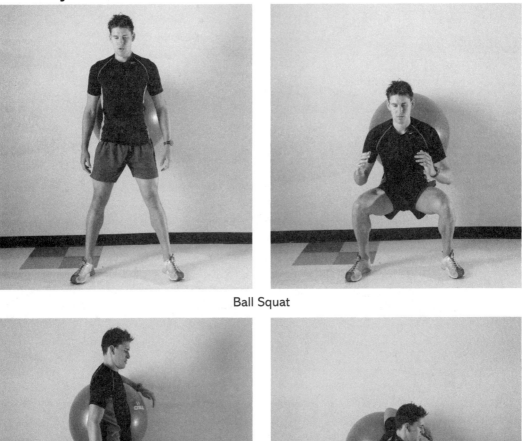

Ball Squat

Ball Single-Leg Squat

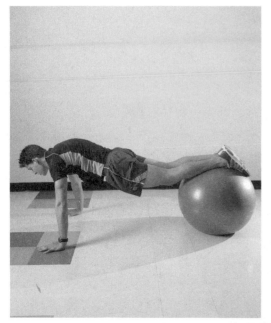
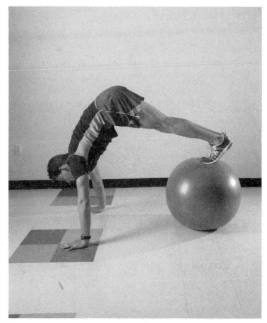

Ball Pike

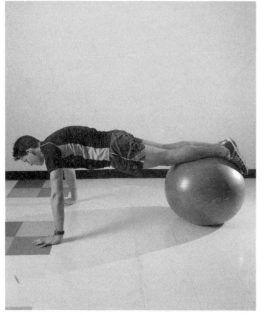
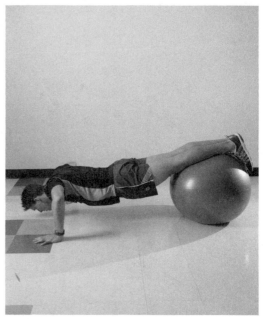

Ball Push-up

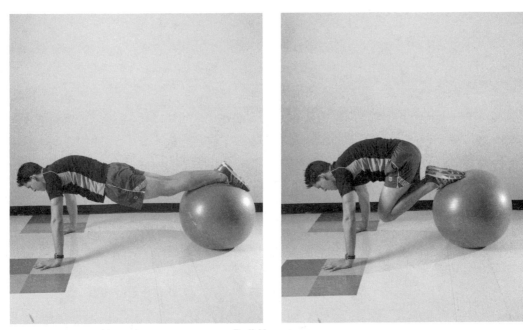

Ball Knee-ups

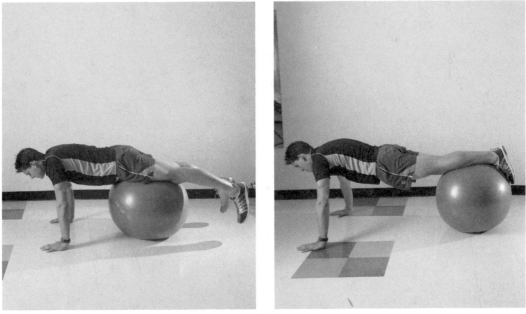

Ball Walkout

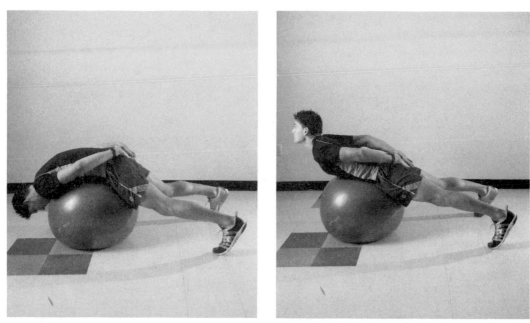

Ball Back Extension

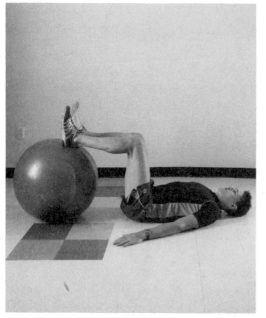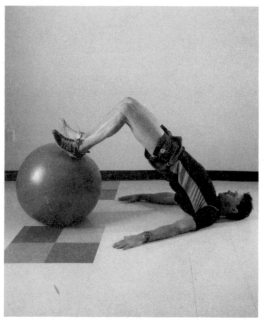

Ball Bridge

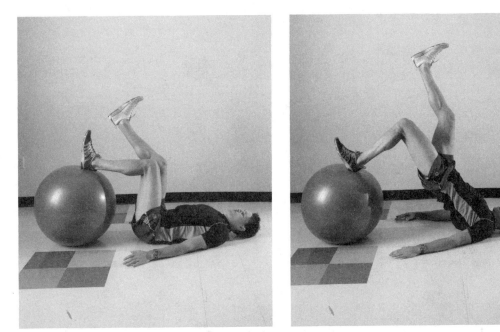

Ball Single-Leg Bridge

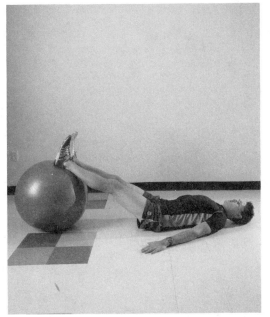
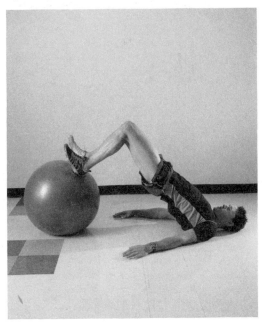

Ball Leg Curls

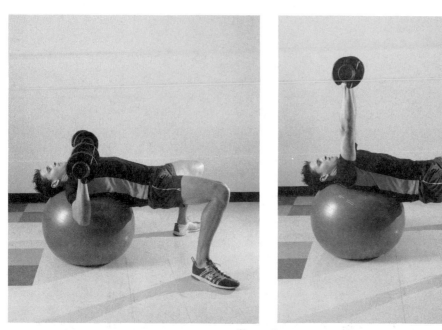

Chest Press

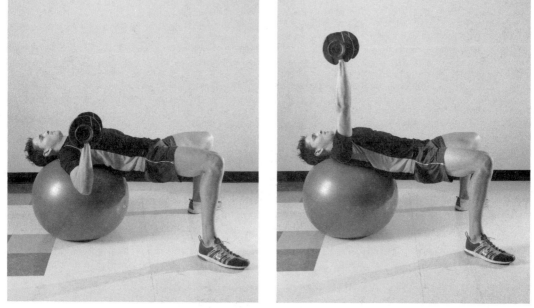

Single-Arm Chest Press

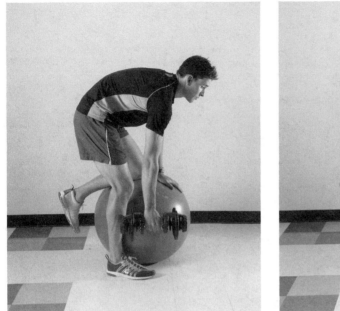 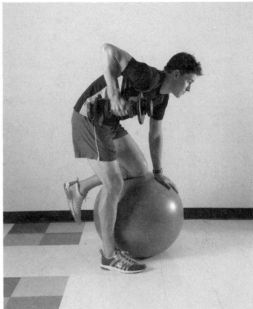

Ball Row

Cables

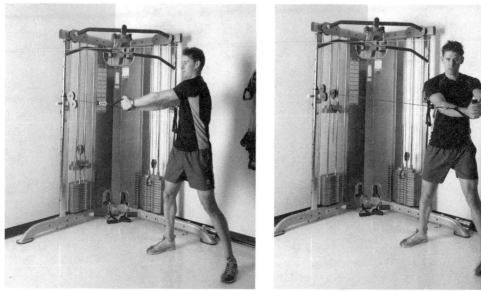

Cable Torso Twist

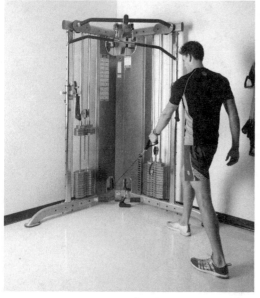
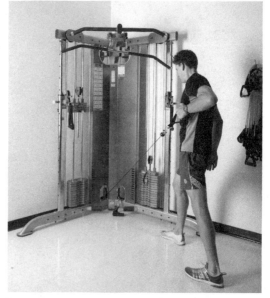

Cable Row

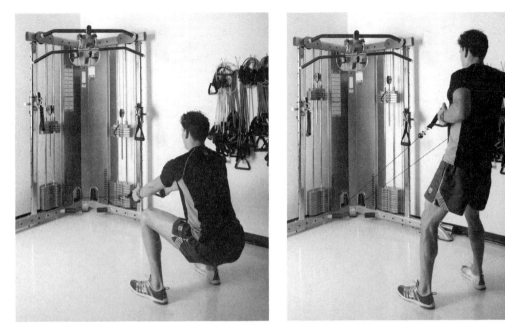

Water-Ski Row

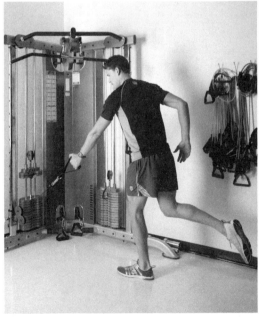
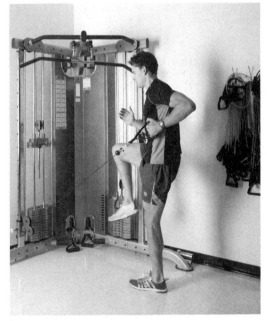

Running Man Row

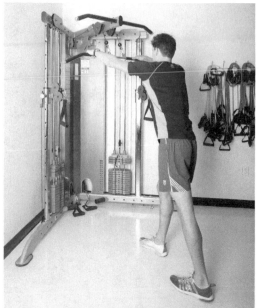 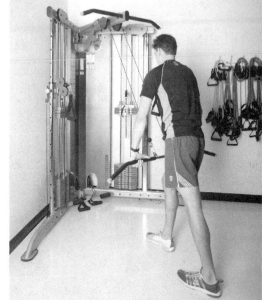

Straight-Arm Cable Pull-downs

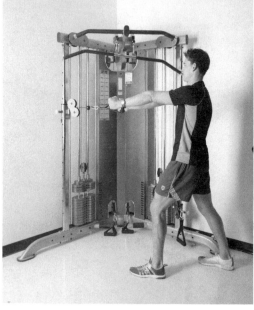 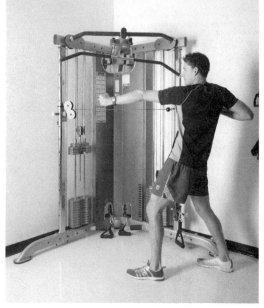

Bow Row

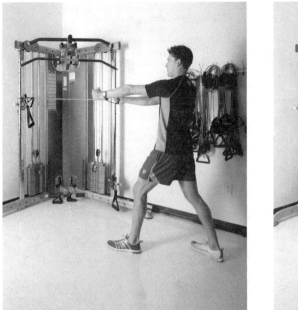 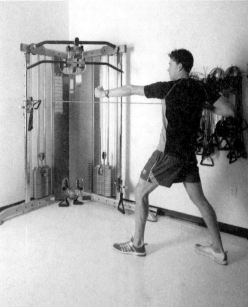

Elastic Band Bow Row

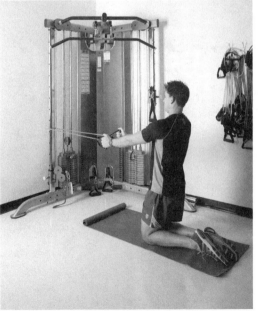 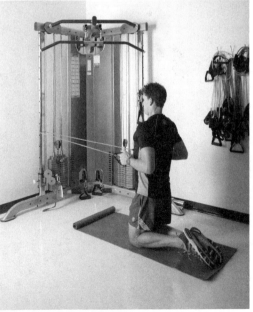

Elastic Band Kneeling Row

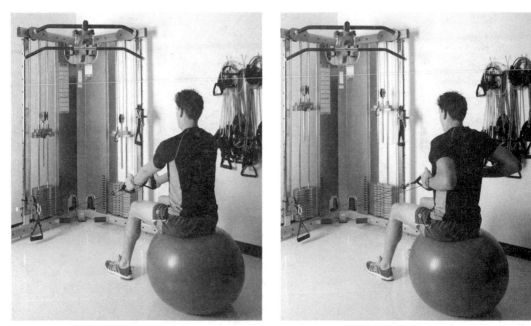

Cable Seated Row

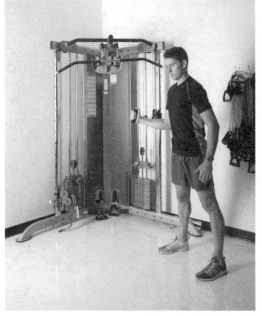
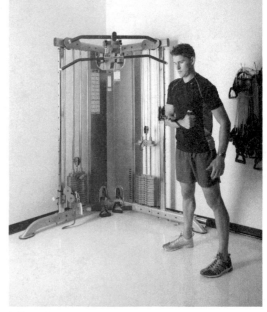

Cable Internal Rotation

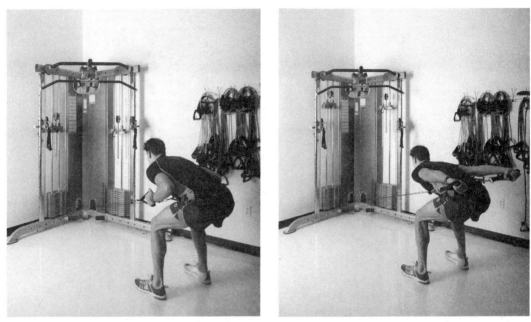

Cable Kickbacks

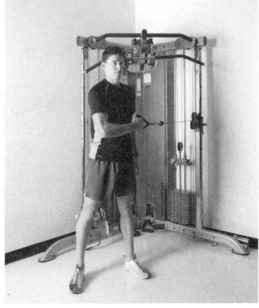 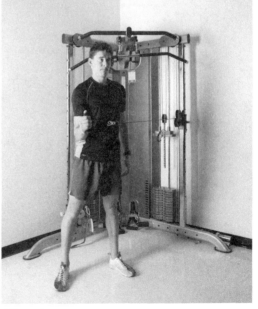

Cable External Rotation

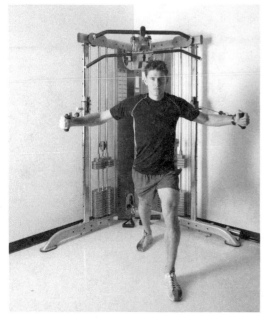 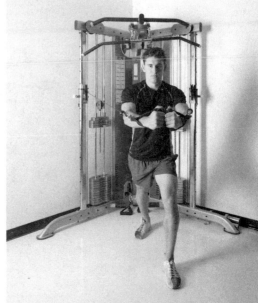

Cable Chest Flies

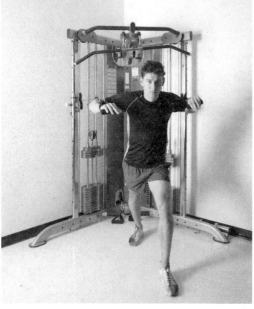 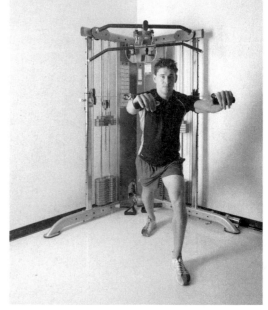

Cable Chest Press

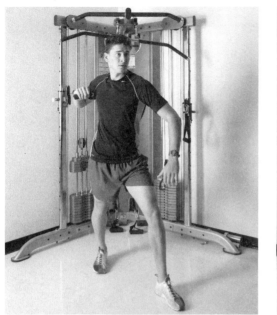
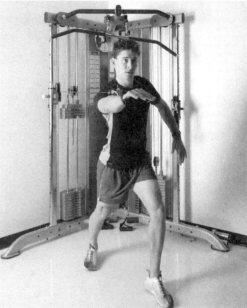

Single-Arm Cable Chest Press

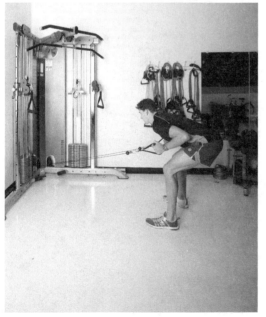
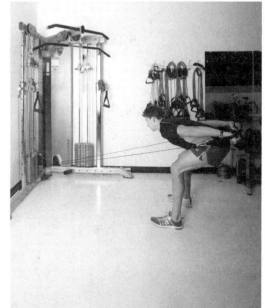

Cable Kickbacks to the Side

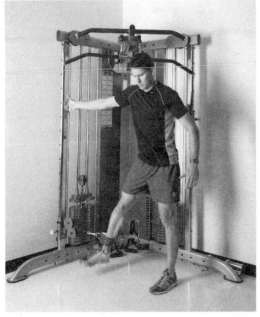 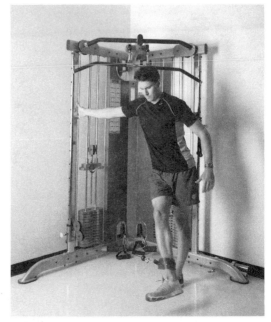

Cable Adduction

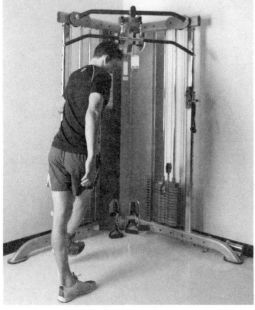 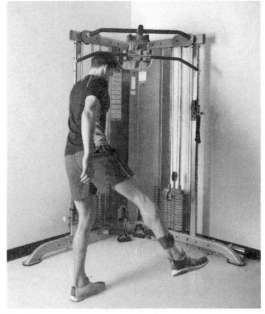

Cable Abduction

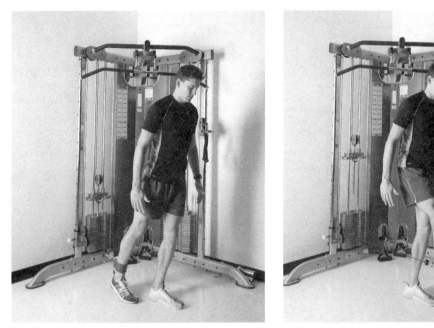

Cable Leg Kickforwards

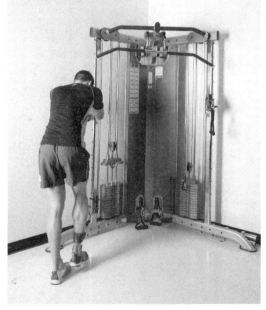 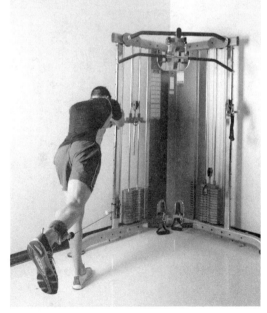

Cable Leg Kickbacks

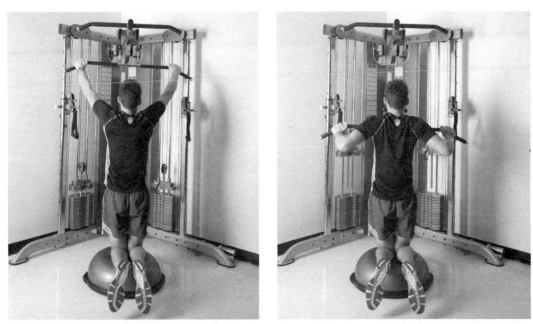

Cable Lat Pull-downs

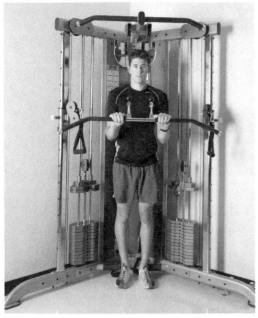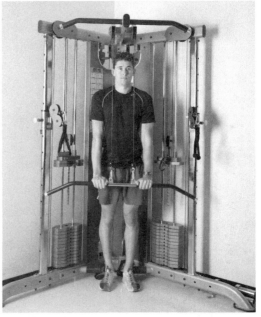

Cable Triceps Push-downs

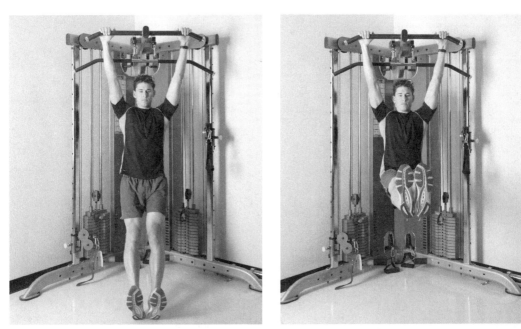

Hanging Straight-Leg Raise

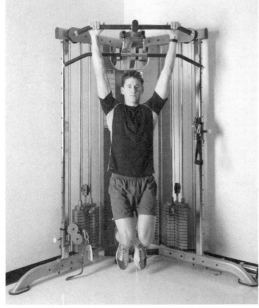
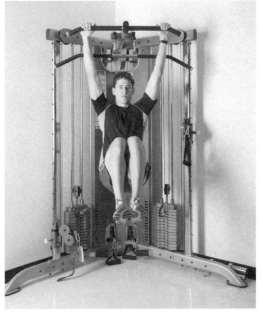

Hanging Bent-Leg Raise

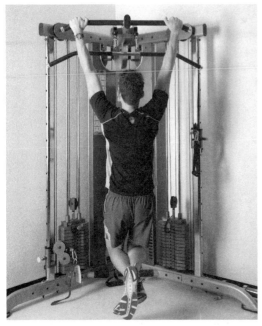
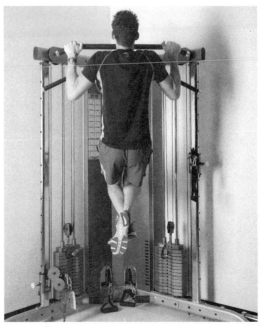

Pull-up

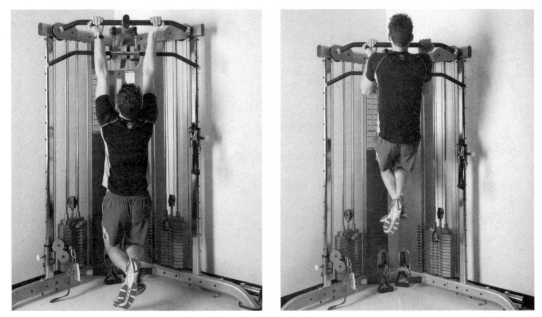

Reverse Grip Pull-up

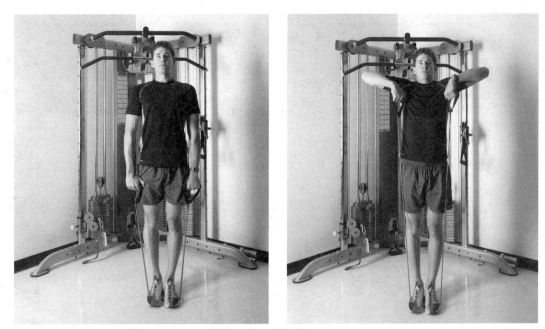

Elastic Band Upright Row

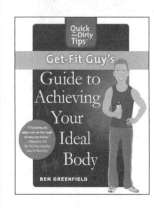
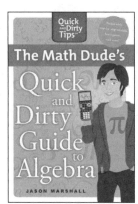
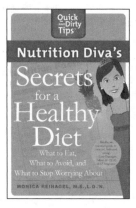
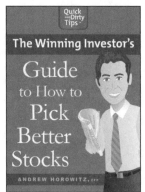
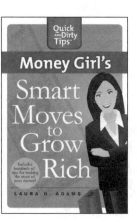
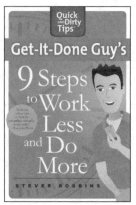